W9-AMM-830

Did You Know That . . .

The herb kudzu may aid in relieving a hangover
and beating alcohol addiction?

Bee propolis (the sticky substance used by bees to seal
their hives) promotes the healing of skin wounds?

The amino acid L-arginine can help you have
better sex and a stronger body?

Guys over fifty can maintain the health of their
prostate by taking the herb saw palmetto?

You do now, thanks to

EARL MINDELL

Also by Earl Mindell, R.Ph., Ph.D.

Earl Mindell's Food as Medicine
Earl Mindell's Secret Remedies
Earl Mindell's Anti-Aging Bible
Earl Mindell's Soy Miracle Cookbook
Earl Mindell's Soy Miracle
Earl Mindell's New Herb Bible
Earl Mindell's Vitamin Bible

Earl Mindell's
SUPPLEMENT
BIBLE

...

Earl Mindell, R.Ph., Ph.D.

POCKET BOOKS

New York   London   Toronto   Sydney   Singapore

The sale of this book without its cover is unauthorized. If you purchased this book without a cover, you should be aware that it was reported to the publisher as "unsold and destroyed." Neither the author nor the publisher has received payment for the sale of this "stripped book."

The ideas, procedures, and suggestions contained in this book are not intended to replace the services of a trained health professional. All matters regarding your health require medical supervision. You should consult your physician before adopting the procedures in this book. Any applications of the treatments set forth in this book are at the reader's discretion.

 POCKET BOOKS, a division of Simon & Schuster, Inc.
1230 Avenue of the Americas, New York, NY 10020

Copyright © 1998 by Earl Mindell, R.Ph., Ph.D., and Carol Colman

Originally published in trade paperback in 1998 by Fireside

All rights reserved, including the right to reproduce this book or portions thereof in any form whatsoever. For information address Fireside, 1230 Avenue of the Americas, New York, NY 10020

ISBN: 0-7432-2661-5

First Pocket Books printing June 2002

10 9 8 7 6 5 4 3 2 1

POCKET and colophon are registered trademarks of Simon & Schuster, Inc.

For information regarding special discounts for bulk purchases, please contact Simon & Schuster Special Sales at 1-800-456-6798 or business@simonandschuster.com

Printed in the U.S.A.

Acknowledgments

I wish to express my deep and lasting appreciation to the people who assisted me on this book, especially Judith Eaton, M.S., R.D., for her wonderful work. Also many thanks to Philip Duterme, president of Ayurvedic Concepts; James H. Zhou, Ph.D., cofounder of HerbaSway; Alan Kratz, Pharm.D., of Homeovits Laboratories; Harold Segal, Ph.D.; Bernard Bubman, R.Ph.; Edward Powell, R.Ph.; Sal Messineo, Pharm.D.; Arnold Fox, M.D.; Dennis Huddleson, M.D.; Rory Jaffe, M.D.; Donald Cruden, O.D.; Nathan Sperling, D.D.S.; and Alan Kashin, R.Ph., Ph.D.

Contents

Introduction

Two decades ago, when I published my first book on supplements, many people considered vitamins (and those of us who took them) a little strange and exotic, and regarded herbs as a useful addition to tomato sauce and nothing more. Now we know that vitamins and herbs can play such an important role in maintaining health and vitality that the overwhelming majority of health-conscious people take supplements daily. In fact, as many as half of all Americans—more than 100 million people—use supplements in one form or another, whether it's a basic multivitamin, a homeopathic remedy for colds and flu, or an herb to treat menopause or prostate problems.

Until recently, however, our choice of supplements was rather limited. For example, many products sold over the counter and used for decades in Europe were simply unavailable in the United States because of restrictive laws. In response to consumer demand, in 1994 Congress passed the Dietary Supplement Health and Education Act (DSHEA), which has radically changed the way supplements are sold and marketed in this country. The law lifted decades of regulatory barriers that had made it difficult, if not impossible, to bring new supplements to market. For one thing, most supplements are derived from natural products, and natural products cannot be patented. Therefore, drug companies are not interested in investing the hundreds of millions of dollars in clinical testing necessary for approval from the Food and Drug Administration (FDA) because they can never recoup their investment. The new law declared supplements to be dietary products and therefore not subject to the rigorous and expensive testing required by the FDA for new drugs. As a result, many supplements that would have been previously classified as drugs and regulated by the FDA can be sold over the counter in health food stores, pharmacies, and even neighborhood grocery stores.

Under the old law, even products that had been used abroad safely for decades could not be sold in the United States without undergoing expensive clinical testing. Under the new law, any product with a reasonable safety record can be quickly brought to market. So, if a product has been used safely for thousands of years by herbal healers, or for decades in other countries without problems, it is no longer necessary for it to undergo the arduous testing procedures required by the FDA. In fact, it is now the responsibility of the FDA to prove that a product is unsafe before it can be pulled off the shelves.

Another major change is that manufacturers are now allowed to make health claims for their products on labels and in advertisements as long as these claims are based on solid, scientific evidence. For example, if a product may help soothe a cold, or prevent osteoporosis, manufacturers are allowed to say so.

The DSHEA has already been a boon to consumers. In 1995 alone, the first year that this law took effect, an astounding *20,000 new supplements* were introduced in the United States. Each year, thousands more are brought to market. A walk through any natural food store or pharmacy dramatically underscores the profound effect this law has already had on the availability of supplements.

In addition to more traditional vitamins, minerals, and herbs that have become household names in recent years, you will also see row upon row of new products with exotic-sounding names. Many of these new products are phytochemicals, extracts of disease-fighting compounds found exclusively in fruits and vegetables, which have only recently been isolated and packaged as supplements. Other new products popping up on the shelves include proteins, amino acids, enzymes, natural hormones (like DHEA and melatonin), and other substances that are produced by the body but that decline as we age and need to be replenished. Still other new supplements are herbs that have been widely used in other countries, but not—until now—in the United States.

The Supplement Bible is the *first* book to introduce readers to the supplement explosion brought about by the recent change in the law. It is written for the tens of millions of supplement users who are bewildered by the avalanche of new products and who are eager to learn about them.

How to Use This Book

At the core of this book are the Hot 100 supplements. Most of the Hot 100 are cutting-edge, "high-tech" supplements that have not before been widely available in the United States. However, within the Hot 100 I have also included some familiar supplements that are now being sold in new and improved forms, or that have lately been the subject of groundbreaking medical news. In each case, I not only tell you about the supplement but show precisely how to use it. Not every supplement is good for everybody; I also caution under what conditions a supplement is not appropriate.

In addition to the Hot 100, 1 have grouped supplements that address specific problems. This makes *The Supplement Bible* especially easy to use if you have a particular need. For example, as of this writing, the diet pills "Phen Fen" have been pulled from the market because of safety concerns. As a result, millions of people are now turning to natural alternatives to help shed extra pounds. I have therefore included a section, "Fat Burners and Sports Supplements," to explain products designed to promote weight loss, build muscle tone, and create a stronger, sleeker body. If your goal is to feel "pumped" or to enhance athletic performance, I have also listed supplements here that will help you achieve those goals.

In addition, I have included special sections on supplements that can help fight depression, jump-start your sex life, make you sharper and smarter, and even rejuvenate your skin. I have also provided the latest information on old favorites, supplements that you may already be taking, as well as a brief guide to homeopathic medicine, which is growing in popularity by leaps and bounds.

ANSWERS TO COMMONLY ASKED QUESTIONS

In addition to writing about health, I also lecture and appear on many talk shows. I am often asked questions about supplements, and I will try to answer some of the most frequently asked questions below.

What is a vitamin?

Vitamins are organic substances that are essential for life and are usually not produced by the body. You must get vitamins from either food or supplements. Vitamins are micronutrients, meaning that you need to ingest a comparatively small amount to function well. If you are severely deficient in a particular vitamin, you will suffer from a deficiency disease. For example, a severe vitamin C deficiency will cause scurvy, and a severe vitamin D deficiency will cause rickets.

There are two kinds of vitamins: water-soluble and fat-soluble. Most vitamins are water-soluble, which means they are not stored in the body and excess amounts are excreted in urine. Fat-soluble vitamins (A, D, E, and K) are stored in fatty tissue. Water-soluble vitamins are measured in micrograms (mcg.) which are $\frac{1}{1,000,000}$ of a gram, or milligrams (mg.) which are $\frac{1}{1000}$ of a gram. Fat-soluble vitamins are measured in IU, international units, with the exception of vitamin A, which is sometimes measured in RE (retinol equivalents): 1 RE = 1 IU.

What is a mineral?

Minerals are naturally occurring chemical elements that are found throughout the body and must be replenished through either food or supplements. They are critical for strong teeth and bones, and for normal cell function. Minerals are divided into two categories: essential minerals and trace minerals. Essential minerals need to be consumed in greater volume and are measured in milligrams or grams. We require only a minuscule amount of trace minerals, and they are measured in micrograms.

What is a nutraceutical?

A nutraceutical is a supplement-enriched food that is designed to protect against various diseases or treat common ailments. Some examples of new nutraceuticals include snack bars fortified with soy phytochemicals to alleviate symptoms such as hot flashes in menopausal women and to prevent prostate problems in men, as well as phytochemical-enriched candy for children who won't eat their vegetables.

What are the RDAs?

The RDAs (Recommended Daily Allowances) are the U.S. government's determinations of the bare minimum amount of certain vitamins and minerals needed to prevent serious deficiency diseases. Compiled decades ago, the RDAs reflect the way medicine is practiced in this country—their focus is on *illness*, not on the maintenance of health and vitality. The RDAs were designed when scientists knew very little about how our cells worked and how micronutrients and cells interact. Today we know that vitamins and minerals do more than protect us from diseases: they play a key role in *preventing* many diseases, including cancer, heart disease, and even depression.

Throughout this book, I cite study after study clearly showing that when blood levels of vitamins, minerals, and other important micronutrients drop below optimal levels, our bodies cannot function properly. For example, the RDA for vitamin E, an essential vitamin for a healthy heart and proper immune function, is a paltry 8 to 10 IU daily; yet, studies sponsored by the U.S. government's own National Institute on Aging show that you need at least 200 IU daily of vitamin E to begin to reap any significant benefit. Periodically, there is talk of revamping the

RDAs to reflect this body of knowledge, but it could be years before anyone gets around to doing it.

Therefore, my dosage recommendations are based not on the RDAs but on the latest scientific studies.

What about supplements that are not included in the RDAs?

The RDAs are only for a select group of vitamins and minerals. They virtually ignore whole categories of important supplements that in recent years have been the subject of numerous research studies. In fact, most of the supplements I write about in this book are not included in the RDAs. For example, there are no RDAs for important compounds found in plants called carotenoids, which include lycopene, lutein, and other phytochemicals that can—among other things—help fight cancer and preserve vision. The importance of carotenoids is underscored by several studies showing that men who eat the most lycopene-rich foods have the lowest rates of prostate cancer. I personally recommend taking a mixed carotenoid supplement to make sure that you are getting enough of these important compounds. Yet, these potentially life-saving compounds are not even mentioned in the RDAs.

The trace mineral chromium picolinate is another example of an important disease-fighting supplement that is excluded from the RDAs. Researchers at the U.S. Department of Agriculture have shown that chromium is an effective treatment for Type II adult-onset diabetes, quite common in the United States, which increases the risk of heart disease. Some 16 million Americans have this problem, and many researchers believe that taking chromium picolinate could help prevent Type II diabetes from occurring in the first place. Yet, there is no mention of chromium in the RDAs. The point is that when a

supplement like chromium is omitted from the RDAs, it
does not mean that it could not be of great benefit to millions of people. All it means is that the RDAs are hope-
lessly outdated.

If you eat a well-balanced diet, do you need to take supplements?

In an ideal world, everyone would be able to eat a "well-
balanced" diet that would eliminate the need for supplements. We would carefully plan out each meal so that we
would have just the right amount of each micronutrient.
But we don't live in an ideal world. Most of us eat on the
run, skip meals, and often choose processed convenience
foods that are nutrient-poor. And although the National
Cancer Institute recommends that people eat five to
eight servings of fruits and vegetables daily, less than 10
percent of the population actually does so. Sadly, on any
given day, 80 to 90 percent of the population is deficient
in one or more of the vitamins and minerals listed in
the RDAs.

I am a great believer in healthy eating and in fact am a
careful eater myself. I eat only fresh food and never touch
junk food. Unlike many folks, I avoid colas with phosphate, which can literally wash minerals out of the body.
I rarely drink alcohol, which can deplete the body of B
vitamins. I don't smoke, which can decrease natural levels of vitamin C. Yet, I know that as careful as I am, I cannot possibly get all the vitamins, minerals, and nutrients I
need from food alone. Even though I try to eat fresh,
organic produce, I am aware that modern farming practices have depleted the soil of nutrients, which in turn
can strip fruits and vegetables of their valuable vitamins
and minerals. The storage and shipping of food can also
sap it of its nutrients. I take supplements to ensure that I

am getting all of the micronutrients I need to maintain optimal health, and I advise others to do the same.

What form of supplement is the most effective?

Supplements come in many different forms, from tablets to capsules to liquids to powders that can be mixed in water or juice to fortified food bars to creams and gels. Choose the form that is easiest for you to use. For example, if you hate to swallow pills, try a liquid extract or powder if it is available. In some cases, however, I do recommend one particular form of a supplement. For example, I recommend the sublingual form of vitamin B_{12} (a tablet that dissolves under the tongue) because it is better absorbed by the body. In other cases, I recommend a particular formulation for a supplement because it is gentler on the stomach.

Is it better to take supplements separately or in combination?

Supplements may be sold separately or as multisupplement combination formulas. For example, as I noted earlier, I recommend taking a mixed carotenoid supplement, which contains several different carotenoids. You can also purchase each carotenoid separately, but obviously it is more convenient to take just one pill. Many different combination formulas are available for specific purposes. For example, there are formulas designed for sleep, weight loss, or better immune function, each of which would include a combination of different herbs, vitamins, and other supplements that should work well together. In some cases, these combination formulas can be a real bargain when compared to the cost of buying each supplement separately. If you use these multisupplement combinations, I advise you to read the labels carefully to make sure that you are getting what you need and that they conform to my recommended dosages. If a multisupplement contains an ingredient you do not want to take, look for a different multisupplement.

When is the best time to take my supplements?

As a rule, most supplements are taken two or three times daily, with meals, unless otherwise specified. In some cases, I will recommend that you take a supplement on an empty stomach, an hour or two before or after eating. For convenience, I advise people to organize their supplements in the morning and to carry what they need with them for the rest of the day in a plastic bag or a pill case.

Supplements that promote sleep or relaxation should be taken only at night before bedtime because they can promote drowsiness. Do not drive or operate any machinery after using these supplements.

There are hundreds of supplements listed in this book; how do I know which ones are for me?

It is not my intention for anyone to take all of the supplements listed in this book, and certainly not all at once. Although some supplements can and should be taken daily, many supplements are to be used just for specific problems, or under specific conditions. For example, there are several wonderful supplements that can help reduce the symptoms of cold and flu, and give your immune system an added boost when you are sick. Once the symptoms disappear, however, you no longer need to take them. Someone suffering from premenstrual syndrome (PMS) may take different supplements from someone looking to relieve menopausal symptoms. If you are a man or woman with high blood lipid levels, which put you at risk of heart disease, or if you are battling the aches and pains of arthritis, you may choose from several supplements that may help relieve your problems.

With so many new supplements on the market, how do I pick a brand that is effective and safe?

The same rules apply to buying supplements that apply to buying any over-the-counter medication: Select products offered by reputable manufacturers that take special steps to ensure safety and effectiveness. You can purchase your supplements in natural food stores, pharmacies, or supermarkets, or through mail order or network marketing companies. Look for products that come in tamper-proof packages, preferably with both an inside and an outside safety seal. Each package should be clearly marked with an expiration date. Also, look for a quality control number on the package; this means that on the off chance something should go awry, the manufacturer can quickly pull the tainted product off the shelf.

In some cases, manufacturers offer products with a guaranteed potency, which means that the product has been analyzed after manufacturing to guarantee the potency stated on the label. Some products may be labeled pharmaceutical grade, which means that they are of the highest quality and are free of impurities.

Although I believe that the overwhelming majority of the supplements sold today are safe, I caution people that just because a product purports to be "natural" and can be obtained without a prescription, it is not necessarily something that can be taken indiscriminately. In fact, as you will see, there are some supplements that I recommend only for certain situations or for very limited use, and even some that I may caution against using at all. When in doubt about taking a supplement, check with your pharmacist, your natural healer, or a knowledgeable physician.

To maintain the maximum effectiveness of your supplements and to retard spoilage, store them in a cool, dark place out of direct sunlight. Some products may need to be refrigerated and will say so on the label.

Is it safe to combine supplements with prescription medication?

It all depends on the supplement. Some supplements, such as Saint John's wort, which is a natural treatment for depression, should not be taken in combination with other antidepressants. In some cases, omega-3 fatty acids, which are natural blood thinners, should not be taken along with prescription blood thinners such as coumadin. Other supplements, however, such as probiotics, are meant to be taken along with prescription antibiotics. My point is that each case is different. In this book, I try to caution when a supplement may interact with another drug or supplement. To be on the safe side, check with your physician or natural healer.

When is it safe to self-medicate with supplements, and when should I call my doctor?

Common sense dictates that you can use supplements to treat the same problems for which you would use any other over-the-counter products. Supplements in particular are good to relieve common ailments such as colds, flu symptoms, sore throats, headaches, stress, and general aches and pains. If you have a high fever or a cold, flu, or sore throat that lasts beyond a few days, or other serious symptoms, you should definitely check with your physician or natural healer. If you have a previously diagnosed medical condition, such as cancer or heart disease, you should also work with a knowledgeable physician who can help you incorporate natural remedies into your regimen.

Before you begin reading *The Supplement Bible*, I want to add one final thought. Supplements are a wonderful way to enhance your health. They can help you maintain your vigor and vitality well into your later years, improve the quality of life, and perhaps even extend your life. As good as they are, supplements cannot do the job alone. Supplements work best when they are supported by a sound diet and a health-conscious lifestyle.

1

The Hot Hundred

FACTS

I kick off the Hot 100 with alpha carotene, first among the illustrious carotenoid family. Carotenoids are substances in fruits and vegetables that are natural coloring agents. Recently, researchers have discovered that carotenoids are much more than mere decoration—they have powerful antioxidant and anticancer properties. Although plants need sunlight to thrive and grow, constant exposure to the ultraviolet (UV) rays emitted by the sun can trigger the formation of dangerous free radicals, which can cause genetic damage. In order to survive, plants need a mechanism to protect themselves from these potentially troublesome UV rays. Carotenoids are natural sunscreens that filter out UV radiation and protect plants and human beings from other environmental carcinogens. There are more than 500 different carotenoids in plants, and about 50 can be found in edible fruits and vegetables.

Of the entire carotenoid family, the most famous is beta carotene. Scientists have primarily focused their research on beta carotene because of its pro-vitamin A activity; that is, it is converted into vitamin A as the body needs it. Until recently, it was widely believed that beta carotene itself was useless and could be used by the body only after its conversion into vitamin A. We now know that carotenoids such as beta carotene may each offer particular advantages. In the 1980s, beta carotene stole the spotlight because of studies that suggested it may protect against certain types of cancer. When researchers investigated whether other carotenoids could also have hidden benefits, the results were quite astonishing. Not only did some of these lesser-known carotenoids show significant anticancer activity, but many were even more potent than beta carotene. A case in point is alpha carotene, long neglected but now a rising star among supplements. Several studies have shown that alpha carotene can drastically reduce the number of tumors in animals with lung, liver, and skin cancer. In fact, alpha carotene may be *ten times* more powerful than beta carotene in protecting skin, eye, liver, and lung tissue against free radical damage. Like beta carotene, alpha carotene is also converted to vitamin A. The best food sources of alpha carotene are cooked carrot and pumpkin.

Alpha carotene is sold alone, included in mixed carotenoid supplements, and included in antioxidant formulas.

POSSIBLE BENEFITS

*Works as a natural antioxidant and free radical scavenger.
Shows strong anticancer activity.*

THE RIGHT AMOUNT

Take 3–6 mg. of mixed carotenoids daily.

Personal Advice

The fruits and vegetables that are commonly eaten in the United States provide about 20 different carotenoids, but Americans often do not get enough carotenoids from diet alone. In fact, studies show that only 10 percent of the population eats five servings of fruits and vegetables daily, as recommended by the National Cancer Institute. Try to eat as many carotenoid-rich foods as possible, such as dark green leafy vegetables, and red and orange fruits. To cover all your bases, however, I recommend taking a broad-spectrum antioxidant with alpha and beta carotenoids, plus two other Hot 100 supplements, lycopene and lutein. (Lycopene has been associated with a reduced risk of prostate cancer; lutein may help protect against macular degeneration.)

L-Arginine

FACTS

Better sex and a stronger body. That's the promise of L-arginine, the natural form of arginine, an amino acid that for obvious reasons is growing more popular with each passing year. Recently, some intriguing new studies have suggested that L-arginine may also enhance immune function and may even be an effective treatment for certain kinds of cancers.

Natural healers recommend L-arginine for men who have problems with sexual function, specifically with maintaining an erection long enough to engage in sex. L-arginine works by increasing blood flow to the penis, which results in harder erections. Alas, the effect is short-lived, so in order to use L-arginine to improve sexual performance, you need to take it about 45 minutes before having sex. Not everyone finds that L-arginine works, but there are enough anecdotal reports by men who have benefited from L-arginine to allow us to take it seriously. Several studies have shown that L-arginine can also increase sperm count and may be a useful treatment for male infertility.

L-arginine is best known for its ability to stimulate the production of growth hormone, which is instrumental in shedding fat and building muscle. Body builders use L-arginine to bulk up and lose flab. L-arginine also has important medical uses. For instance, it is used in hospitals to promote wound healing in patients after surgery, and for those suffering from severe burns.

According to several studies, L-arginine can boost immune function by stimulating the thymus gland, a tiny gland that sits behind the breastbone. The thymus gland is where important disease-fighting cells called T-lymphocytes (T-cells) are stored until they are called into action to defend the body against infection. Studies show that L-arginine can increase the number of T-cells, enabling the body to protect itself better against unwanted microorganisms. Several Japanese researchers have shown that in test tube studies, L-arginine in combination with human immune cells can also trigger the production of natural killer cells, one of the body's defenses against cancer. Animal studies show that L-arginine can inhibit the growth of many different types of cancerous tumors. Because of studies such as these, researchers are studying the use of L-arginine as a potential cancer treatment.

POSSIBLE BENEFITS

Enhances sexual performance in men.
May help to build muscle.
Boosts immune function.

THE RIGHT AMOUNT

For its sex-enhancing benefits, take 3–6 grams of L-arginine on an empty stomach 45 minutes before having sex.

CAUTIONS

Although there is no solid evidence to confirm it, some researchers believe that arginine may trigger the onset of herpes infection. However, this may be avoided by taking it with 500 mg. of lysine, which can inhibit the herpes virus.

Ashwagandha (*Withania somnifera*)

FACTS

Known as Indian ginseng, this herb is derived from the roots and leaves of the *Withania somnifera* shrub and is part of the traditional Ayurvedic system of medicine. In the West, researchers have focused on isolating the one or two active ingredients within each herb. In the Ayurvedic tradition, however, the entire plant is used on the assumption that all the compounds in a plant are meant to work together. For more than 1,000 years, ashwagandha has been highly prized as a treatment for impotence, stress, infertility, and arthritis. Because of its wide range of activity in many different body systems, ashwagandha is reputed to be an overall tonic that can promote health and vitality, much like ginseng (see page 184). Also like ginseng, ashwagandha is reputed to increase stamina, physical performance, and mental acuity. The concept of tonic herbs is difficult to describe in Western terms because we do not have anything comparable in our system of medicine. In general, tonics such as ashwagandha are believed to strengthen and fortify the body so that it is better able to withstand stressful situations. In other words, these herbs help the body to maintain its equilibrium, even during difficult times.

Today, ashwagandha is included in many combination formulas of Ayurvedic herbs to treat a variety of ills. In particular, ashwagandha is now being heavily promoted as an aphrodisiac and sex-enhancing supplement. It is sold in combination with other herbal supplements that are reputed to improve sexual desire and function, such as puncturevine (tribulus). Ayurvedic healers say that ashwagandha can improve sex drive and the ability to maintain an erection.

A natural anti-inflammatory agent, ashwagandha may help to reduce the discomfort associated with arthritis. One study conducted at the University of Poona in Poona, India, reported that when given an herbal formula combining ashwagandha and zinc complex, patients reported a significant reduction in pain and stiffness. There are several Ayurvedic antiarthritic formulas on the market; many include boswellia, another Hot 100 herb (see page 13).

POSSIBLE BENEFITS

Enhances energy.
Improves sexual performance.
Relieves arthritis.

THE RIGHT AMOUNT

Take up to three 4.5-mg. standardized tablets daily.

Bee Propolis

FACTS

Bee propolis (also known as bee glue) is the sticky substance used by bees to seal their hives to protect them from unwanted intruders and infection. Insects or small animals who haplessly enter the hive are first stung to death and then embalmed with propolis to prevent disease-causing decay. Bees don't make propolis; they gather it from trees. Propolis includes many different substances, such as resins, vitamins, minerals, and a large amount of bioflavonoids. Propolis, the Greek word for "defender of the city," was highly valued in ancient times. Early healers intuitively knew that propolis was a natural disinfectant, and they used it for a wide variety of ailments. Hippocrates prescribed it to heal skin wounds and soothe angry stomach ulcers. The great English herbalist Nicholas Culpeper wrote that propolis was "good for all heat and inflammation in many parts of the body and cools the heat of the wounds." During both world wars, soldiers applied propolis to their wounds to prevent infection.

Intrigued by the folklore, modern scientists investigated propolis and discovered that it does indeed have natural antibiotic, antiviral, and anti-inflammatory compounds. Recent trials conducted at the National Heart and Lung Institute confirmed that propolis is effective against a wide range of disease-producing microbes, including *Staphylococcus aureus* MRSA, commonly known as staph, which is resistant to most antibiotics and is common in hospitals. This is particularly important, considering that the overuse of antibiotics is creating a new breed of "monster" bacteria that is resistant to all known antibiotics. If we are to stop the spread of drug-resistant bacteria, we must look to new types of natural therapies like propolis that can keep bacteria in check.

Propolis can be used both externally and internally. Recently, natural healers have found that propolis is an excellent treatment for sore gums, mouth ulcers, and sore throats. Propolis salve can be rubbed on sore gums to soothe inflammation and prevent infection. As a gargle, propolis can help relieve the pain of sore throat and mouth ulcers and promote healing. Propolis is effective against the herpes virus; when gently applied to the herpes lesion, propolis can help relieve pain. When taken orally in capsule form, propolis is reputed to stimulate immune function.

POSSIBLE BENEFITS

Promotes healing of skin wounds.
Treats sore throats and gum disease.

THE RIGHT AMOUNT

Take one 200-mg. capsule daily.

Personal Advice

At the first sign of cold symptoms, I dissolve a zinc lozenge in my mouth and take vitamin C, propolis, echinacea, and goldenseal. By the next day, the cold disappears.

Beta-1,3 Glucan

FACTS

When I was training to be a pharmacist in the 1960s, I was taught that infectious diseases were a thing of the past. Dazzled by the discovery of so-called wonder drugs like penicillin and the other antibiotics that followed, we believed that there were no diseases that couldn't be cured by simply swallowing a few pills. We now know that we were mistaken. Although antibiotics have saved countless lives, they are not the panacea we once believed them to be. First, they are ineffective against viruses. Second, because of the overuse of antibiotics (discussed in the section on bee propolis), we have created strains of antibiotic-resistant bacteria. There has been a growing acknowledgment by medical professionals that the key to beating disease is to avoid getting sick in the first place, and the best way to ensure good health is to maintain a strong and effective immune system.

Beta-1,3 glucan is one supplement that can help achieve those goals. It is extracted from the cell walls of baker's yeast and is a potent immune enhancer. Specifically, it activates important immune cells, called macrophages, which are often referred to as the "PAC-MAN" of the immune system. Macrophages circulate throughout the body, gobbling up viruses, bacteria, fungi, cancer cells, and other potentially harmful invaders. In addition, the activation of macrophages turns on other components of the immune system that defend us against illness. By fortifying the immune system, beta-1,3 glucan helps weed out troublemakers before they can make us sick.

Beta-1,3 glucan is also an antioxidant: it can protect against free radical damage due to radiation exposure, which is very important because we are all exposed to radiation in one form or another. For example, sunlight is a major source of UV radiation, which not only can cause skin cancer but can severely depress immune function and lead to serious health problems. Every time we are x-rayed, we are exposed to low levels of radiation. In addition, radiation therapy is often used as a cancer treatment. Studies performed by the U.S. Armed Forces Radiobiology Institute showed that beta-1,3 glucan can provide powerful protection against radiation damage. After being exposed to a lethal dose of radiation, rats were given beta-1,3 glucan for 20 days following exposure. Normally, after being exposed to such high doses of radiation, rats, like humans, would develop radiation sickness, which can be fatal. However, 90 percent of the rats that had been given the beta-1,3 glucan were completely protected against radiation damage. Notably, beta-1,3 glucan appeared to have a strong protective effect on immune function, which may explain why the rats remained healthy.

Alternative medicine physicians are now recommending beta-1,3 glucan to their patients with chronic infections, such as *Candida albicans*, Epstein-Barr virus, herpes, and even HIV. Beta-1,3 glucan not only is being used by the chronically ill but is becoming popular among competitive athletes. Ironically, even though exercise is beneficial in many ways, the physical stress of a strenuous workout can dampen immune function. That is why marathon runners are especially vulnerable to respiratory infections after an intensive training period. Some physicians also recommend immune-enhancing supplements such as beta-1,3 glucan to older patients who are experiencing the normal age-related decline in immune function.

Not only can beta-1,3 glucan improve immune function, it can lower high cholesterol and triglyceride levels as well as some prescription medications can, but without the side effects. High cholesterol and triglyceride levels are risk factors for heart disease and stroke.

POSSIBLE BENEFITS

Strengthens immune function.
Protects against radiation damage.
Reduces high blood lipid levels.

THE RIGHT AMOUNT

Take one 2.5-mg. capsule daily 30 minutes before a meal,
or at least 2 hours after eating.

Bilberry

FACTS

Bilberry, also known as European blueberry, is the herb that is synonymous with healthy eyes. For more than 1,000 years, bilberry has been a folk remedy for a variety of eye problems. In fact, during World War II, Royal Air Force pilots ate bilberry jam before night missions to improve their vision. Bilberry contains compounds called anthocyanosides, natural antioxidants that protect the capillaries (small blood vessels) from free radical damage, thereby improving circulation. Anthocyanosides are also involved in the regeneration of a retinal pigment needed to help the eye adapt to light. Bilberry may be beneficial to people suffering from many different forms of eye disease, including glaucoma, which is caused by high ocular pressure, and diabetic retinopathy, which results from poor circulation to the eye. In fact, anthocyanosides derived from bilberry are included in most combination products designed to enhance and protect vision. A prescription medicine (Myrtocyan R) is produced from bilberry extract, providing yet another example of the enormous debt that modern medicine owes to nature's pharmacy.

Although bilberry does not cure these problems, it may help prevent further damage by improving blood flow to the eyes.

Recent research reveals that this remarkable herb is not only good for your eyes but may be useful in the prevention and treatment of other vascular conditions. When circulation is poor, it can hamper the flow of blood to the legs and feet, resulting in pain, numbness, tingling of the skin, and fluid retention. Several studies have shown that anthocyanosides can help relieve these potentially debilitating symptoms. If you have these problems, it is essential to work with a physician to develop the right treatment regimen for you.

There's still more good news about bilberry. In 1996, researchers discovered that bilberry extract shows anti-carcinogenic activity. More studies are needed to determine whether bilberry, like so many other herbs, will prove to be useful in the prevention and treatment of cancer.

POSSIBLE BENEFITS

Protects against common vision problems.
Improves circulation.

THE RIGHT AMOUNT

Bilberry is available in capsules and liquid extract. Take up to three 500-mg. capsules daily. If you prefer to use the liquid extract, take 10 drops in water or juice up to three times daily.

Personal Advice

Bilberry works best when combined with vitamin C. (Take up to 500 mg. vitamin C complex.)

Boswellia

FACTS

Boswellia is one of several ancient herbal remedies that is now on the cutting edge of alternative medicine. Used for thousands of years in the Ayurvedic medical system in India, boswellia is being rediscovered as a treatment for osteoarthritis (so-called wear-and-tear arthritis) and rheumatoid arthritis (RA), an autoimmune disorder that causes the destruction of cartilage, the protective covering that cushions bones. Rheumatoid arthritis can cause pain and swelling in the joints and, in severe cases, can be debilitating. There is no cure for either type of arthritis, although they are commonly treated with nonsteroidal anti-inflammatory drugs (NSAIDs). The problem is that all of these drugs can cause side effects, notably gastric problems, such as ulcers. In addition, most people find that the beneficial effects of these drugs are short-lived; as a result, they need to switch medications frequently.

Natural remedies such as boswellia can relieve arthritis without the potentially dangerous side effects of NSAIDs. In studies of arthritis patients, boswellia has produced some impressive results and was as effective in treating pain and inflammation as one of the most frequently prescribed NSAIDs. Boswellia blocks the synthesis of leukotrienes, substances in the body that can trigger inflammation and promote the formation of free radicals. It may also be useful for the treatment of other inflammatory conditions, such as psoriasis and ulcerative colitis.

Several antiarthritis formulas combine boswellia along with other anti-inflammatory Ayurvedic herbs, including curcumin (see page 42) and ashwagandha (see page 5).

At the same time boswellia relieves arthritis, it also helps prevent heart disease. According to Indian studies, boswellia can lower high blood levels of cholesterol and triglyceride, two risk factors for heart disease and stroke.

POSSIBLE BENEFITS

Relieves symptoms of arthritis.
Normalizes blood lipid levels.

THE RIGHT AMOUNT

Boswellia is available in capsules and topical cream. Take three 500-mg. capsules daily. Once symptoms subside, reduce dose to one 500-mg. capsule daily.

Gently massage boswellia cream into affected areas up to three times daily. Do not use on children under 2 years of age without consulting with a health care practitioner.

Bovine Tracheal Cartilage

FACTS

More than two decades ago, John Prudden, M.D., Med.Sci.D., then an associate professor of clinical surgery at Columbia Presbyterian Medical Center, reported that bovine tracheal cartilage not only promoted the rapid healing of wounds but could cause breast tumors to shrink. Amazed at what he had discovered, Dr. Prudden performed many other studies on bovine tracheal cartilage. Thanks to his work and the work of others who followed, we now know that bovine tracheal cartilage is powerful medicine. In fact, the U.S. Food and Drug Administration recently granted investigational new drug status (IND) to bovine tracheal cartilage to allow researchers at the Cancer Treatment Centers of America to test it on patients who have not responded to either chemotherapy or radiation. Earlier studies on bovine tracheal cartilage, performed in the U.S. and abroad, have reported positive results with many cancer patients. In fact, according to Dr. Prudden's studies, bovine tracheal cartilage cured patients for whom other treatments were ineffective. Unlike chemotherapy or radiation, which work by killing cancer cells but often at the expense of healthy cells, bovine tracheal cartilage stimulates the body's own immune system so that it can successfully ward off the cancer. When used along with chemotherapy or radiation, bovine tracheal cartilage can ameliorate some of the potentially debilitating side effects of these treatments.

Bovine tracheal cartilage is also a very effective treatment for arthritis, a common condition caused by the destruction of cartilage, the protective covering that cushions bone and protects it from injury. More than half of all people over 65 suffer from some form of arthritis, and many take nonsteroidal anti-inflammatory drugs (NSAIDs) to control their pain. Unfortunately, the effects of NSAIDs are often short-lived, and even if they work, they can cause serious side effects, such as bleeding ulcers. Bovine tracheal cartilage may be a safe alternative to NSAIDs for many people. Numerous researchers have reported that bovine tracheal cartilage can lessen the pain and inflammation typical of arthritis. Even better, it is nontoxic and does not cause undesirable side effects.

POSSIBLE BENEFITS

Treats cancer with or without conventional therapy.
Relieves discomfort of arthritis.

THE RIGHT AMOUNT

Take up to three 750-mg. capsules daily.

Personal Advice

If bovine tracheal cartilage alone does not help your arthritic symptoms, try using it in combination with 500 mg. of shark cartilage.

Broccoli Isolates (Extracts)

FACTS

"Eat your vegetables, or no dessert!" If you were the kind of kid who was perfectly willing to forgo dessert as long as you didn't have to eat your veggies, and if even today you can't stomach the thought of broccoli, kale, and other cruciferous vegetables, you're in good company. About 25 percent of the population has an inherited aversion to the bitter taste of cruciferous vegetables. Researchers have dubbed these people "supertasters" because they are highly sensitive to certain flavors. Because of self-imposed dietary limitations, most supertasters do not get all the beneficial phytochemicals from their food that they need to maintain optimum health. Only 10 percent of all Americans actually eat the five servings daily of fruits and vegetables as recommended by the National Cancer Institute, and in all likelihood, few supertasters even come close to meeting this goal.

What are these supertasters missing? Cruciferous vegetables are chock-full of several important cancer-fighting compounds, including indoles, natural free radical scavengers that can deactivate potential carcinogens. In addition, indoles can weaken potent estrogens which can promote the growth of estrogen-sensitive breast tumors. Cruciferous vegetables also contain another powerful anti-cancer compound, sulforaphane, which stimulates the body to produce cancer-fighting enzymes. Not surprisingly, vegetarians have lower rates of nearly every type of cancer than do people who don't eat as many vegetables. The good news is that many of the beneficial substances found in cruciferous vegetables have been extracted from broccoli and are now available in pills or capsules. I'm not suggesting that swallowing a pill is as beneficial as eating a plate of fresh vegetables; vegetables contain fiber and other good things that may not find their way into a supplement. I do believe, however, that broccoli isolates offer many of the advantages of the whole vegetable and are a good alternative for people who do not eat these vegetables anyway.

POSSIBLE BENEFITS

Can inhibit the formation of cancerous tumors.

THE RIGHT AMOUNT

I take a combination supplement of 52 vegetables and fruits that is a wonderful pick-me-up between meals and ensures that I get enough of these valuable phytochemicals. Look for a supplement that contains broccoli isolates or extracts.

Personal Advice

Usually I advise people to steer clear of the salt shaker; however, I'll make this one exception. If you find the taste of broccoli to be too bitter for your liking, try flavoring it with some salt. Some people find that the salty flavor neutralizes the bitter cruciferous flavor. But if you have high blood pressure, do not salt your food.

Bromelain

FACTS

Bromelain, an enzyme derived from pineapple juice, has powerful anti-inflammatory and protein-digesting properties. An excellent digestive aid, bromelain enhances the absorption of nutrients from foods and supplements. Bromelain can also be taken to reduce pain and inflammation following injury, and in at least one respect it offers a decided advantage over nonsteroidal anti-inflammatory drugs (NSAIDs) such as ibuprofen and naprosyn. Such drugs work by inhibiting prostaglandins, hormone-like compounds that can cause inflammation in many parts of the body. Paradoxically, prostaglandins actually have a protective effect on the stomach lining, which is why NSAIDs can cause problems ranging from mild stomach upset to the more serious bleeding ulcers. In contrast, bromelain blocks inflammation by stimulating the production of plasmin, a compound in the body that breaks down fibrinogen, a substance involved in localized swelling. Although bromelain works well in reducing pain and inflammation, it does so without the gastrointestinal distress typical of NSAIDs.

Bromelain is also growing in popularity among athletes who suffer frequent wear-and-tear injuries. Because of its effect on fibrinogen, bromelain may also prevent an even more serious problem: blood clots. Fibrinogen is necessary for the proper clotting of blood so that we don't bleed to death when we are injured, but abnormally high levels of fibrinogen can cause blood clots to form spontaneously, which can lead to a heart attack or stroke. In fact, high levels of fibrinogen have been associated with an increased risk of heart disease.

Smokers have higher than normal levels of fibrinogen and are at greater risk of having a heart attack. In one study of patients with heart disease, bromelain was shown to break down fibrinogen and prevent blood cells from sticking together. According to another German study, a dose of 1000 to 1400 mg. per day of bromelain helped to completely relieve angina, or chest pain, in 14 heart patients. Some patients saw results in as quickly as three days; others, within 90 days. If you have a history of heart disease, you may want to talk to your physician or natural healer about adding this supplement to your daily regimen. Bromelain is also included in many formulas for cardiovascular health.

POSSIBLE BENEFITS

Aids digestion.
Reduces swelling and pain due to inflammation.
Prevents blood clots.

THE RIGHT AMOUNT

To aid digestion, take one or two tablets after meals.
To reduce inflammation, take up to three 500-mg. tablets daily.
For cardiovascular health, take one 500-mg. tablet daily.

Personal Advice

Look for "Gelatin Digestion Unit" (GDU) on the label (450–600 GDU should be stated on the label).

Cat's Claw (Uña de Gato)

FACTS

Practically overnight, this once obscure herb, native to South and Central America, has leaped to fame, primarily because of its reputation for strengthening the immune system. More than four dozen brands of cat's claw products are now prominently displayed in natural food stores throughout the United States.

The cat's claw story is a fascinating one because it underscores many of the problems involved in getting funding for herbal research. For centuries, herbal healers in Peru and other Latin American countries have used cat's claw to treat health problems ranging from arthritis to cancer to intestinal disorders. In the 1970s, cat's claw made headlines around the world when several well-known Peruvians—including a popular actor and a government official—publicly announced that this herb had cured their cancers. These anecdotal success stories attracted the attention of the National Cancer Institute, which tested several compounds from this plant against leukemia cells. The early results were very promising, but because of a lack of funding, research was halted, at least in this country. Since herbs cannot be patented, pharmaceutical companies have little interest in supporting this research because they will not be able to recoup their investment.

Nevertheless, research continued outside the United States, primarily in Europe and Latin America. Periodically, new and exciting information was revealed about cat's claw. In 1991, researchers discovered that cat's claw contained a natural anti-inflammatory agent, and this discovery confirmed its reputation as a treatment for arthritis. Cat's claw was back in the news again in 1993, when European researchers reported the results of a study in which HIV-positive patients were given standardized cat's claw root extract. As you probably know, the AIDS virus knocks out the body's own disease-fighting T-cells, and anything that can boost T-cells is nothing short of miraculous. Fourteen patients participated in the study, which lasted six years. Five of the patients were symptom-free at the beginning of the study, and amazingly, they stayed that way. The other patients, who had experienced some symptoms at the beginning of the study, showed improvement during the first year of treatment with cat's claw. What was truly remarkable was that during the first two and a half years of the study, their T-cell count increased, which indicated that their immune systems were getting stronger. After that, the T-cells reached a plateau.

While cat's claw is certainly not a cure for AIDS, researchers expressed cautious optimism that it may help extend the lives of AIDS patients. Needless to say, there was a run on cat's claw, and shortly thereafter signs began to appear in the windows of natural food stores: "We have cat's claw." As much as I like to see an herb finally get the recognition it deserves, I must point out that even the most ardent supporters of cat's claws are quick to say that more research needs to be done before it can be proclaimed a treatment for AIDS or cancer. However, we can safely say that this herb does appear to bolster immune function, which can help the body fight against infections of all kinds—perhaps even cancer. In addition, I have heard numerous anecdotal reports from people with arthritis who claimed that cat's claw has helped relieve their symptoms. Since cat's claw is nontoxic and safe, at least at recommended doses, there is certainly no harm in trying it.

POSSIBLE BENEFITS

Enhances immune function.
Reduces pain and inflammation associated with arthritis.
May help prevent or treat cancer.

THE RIGHT AMOUNT

Take up to three 500-mg. capsules daily.

Cetyl Myristoleate

FACTS

Cetyl myristoleate (CM) is a new natural treatment for arthritis that is getting good reviews by users, although there are few clinical studies of it. Cetyl myristoleate was discovered in the 1970s by Harry W. Diehl, a researcher at the National Institute of Arthritis, Metabolic and Digestive Diseases, who was reportedly seeking an effective treatment for a friend who suffered from a particularly debilitating case of arthritis. Diehl noticed that one breed of mouse used in the laboratory—the Swiss albino mouse—did not get arthritis even when it was exposed to a particular microorganism that normally causes arthritis in animals. Diehl suspected that the Swiss albino mice had some kind of inborn protection—an arthritic protective factor—which prevented them from developing arthritis. He hoped that if he identified this mysterious antiarthritic substance it would also work on humans.

Diehl eventually isolated CM, a fatty acid that occurs in small amounts in foods such as nuts, vegetables, and butter and in many different species of animals. Swiss albino mice have unusually high levels of this fatty acid. In a fascinating experiment, Diehl tested CM on laboratory rats that he infected with Freud's adjutant, an arthritis-causing agent. Two groups of rats were injected with the arthritis-causing agent, but one group was also given CM. Predictably, the group that did not receive the CM developed arthritis, but amazingly, the group that was given CM remained arthritis free.

Since CM is nontoxic, Diehl gave it to family members and friends with arthritis who found that it worked well in controlling their arthritic symptoms. In 1991, Diehl developed a commercial brand of CM for osteoarthritis, sold primarily through mail order. Other brands of CM are now being brought to market. As of this writing, there are no double-blind clinical studies of CM, and most of the positive reports of it are purely anecdotal. Even its most ardent proponents admit that it does not work for everyone, but then again, neither does any arthritis treatment. Typically, arthritis sufferers have to try several different treatments until they find one that works for them. You can add CM to the list of supplements that may help, though, or take it along with other antiarthritic supplements.

POSSIBLE BENEFITS

Relieves symptoms of arthritis.

THE RIGHT AMOUNT

Each brand of CM has its own treatment protocol. The usual dose is three to five capsules daily for up to one month, depending on the amount of CM in each capsule. The treatment may be repeated several times a year as needed.

CAUTION

CM is most effective for people who avoid alcohol, carbonated beverages, and a high-sugar diet.

Chitosan

FACTS

Chitosan is a "fat blocker," a supplement that enhances weight loss by preventing the absorption of fat. Derived from chitin, which is found in the exoskeletons of shellfish such as shrimp and crabs, chitosan is similar to plant fiber in that it is not digested by the body. When taken orally, chitosan acts like a "fat sponge." As it passes through the digestive tract it can absorb four to six times its weight in fat, thereby flushing it out of the body before it can be metabolized and stored as excess pounds. In other words, you can have your cake and eat it too—as long as you use chitosan!

Alas, chitosan is not a cure for chronic overeating. It should only be used occasionally—perhaps as a tool to "jump-start" a diet, and not for more than two weeks at a time. The problem is that while chitosan is chasing the fat out of your body it can also rob you of fat-soluble vitamins, such as vitamins E, A, D, and K. Therefore, I cannot recommend it for long-term use. If you are taking chitosan, you must supplement your diet with fat-soluble vitamins and essential fatty acids. Otherwise, chitosan appears to be safe, and some studies suggest that it may even be beneficial beyond its potential as a weight-loss tool. For example, one recent study showed that when mice were fed a known carcinogen, the mice eating a chitosan-supplemented diet had fewer precancerous lesions of the colon than the mice not given chitosan. Studies have also shown that chitosan can dramatically lower total blood cholesterol levels and raise the levels of HDL, or good cholesterol, which protects against heart disease. This versatile supplement is also reputed to prevent tooth decay and is an excellent antacid.

POSSIBLE BENEFITS

Can help promote weight loss by blocking absorption of fat.

Lowers cholesterol levels.

May protect against colon cancer.

THE RIGHT AMOUNT

Take up to three 250-mg. tablets daily with meals. Be sure to drink 8 ounces of clear filtered water with each tablet.

CAUTIONS

Do not use chitosan if you have an allergy to shellfish. This supplement (or any other fat blocker) should not be used by pregnant or lactating women or by children.

GENERAL ADVICE

If you are taking chitosan, or any other fiber supplement, be sure to drink at least 8 glasses of water daily.

Chitosan works best when combined with a sensible diet and exercise regimen.

Chlorella

FACTS

Chlorella (*Chlorella pyrenoidosa*) is an edible, single-celled plant that lives in fresh water. Characterized as a "green food," a group of food products derived from other microalgae, chlorella is packed with important phytochemicals that have unique disease-fighting properties, as well as amino acids, vitamins, and minerals. Widely used in Japan, chlorella is touted as the supplement that can help remove or "detoxify" harmful chemicals, heavy metals, and pollutants from the body. Natural healers recommend chlorella for nonspecific complaints such as fatigue and for anyone who generally wants to feel stronger or healthier. It is also used by alternative physicians as part of an overall cancer treatment program.

Japanese researchers recently discovered that chlorella can raise blood levels of the protein albumin. Albumin is one of the body's most powerful antioxidants as well as its main transport system, carrying vitamins, minerals, fatty acids, hormones, and other essential substances throughout the body. Albumin is also instrumental in carrying toxins away from cells and into the liver, where they are broken down and later excreted from the body. Without adequate levels of albumin, the kidneys, liver, and other vital organs cannot do their jobs as well, and the immune system cannot function as efficiently. Numerous studies have documented that a low albumin level is a marker for serious illnesses such as cancer and heart disease. This finding is underscored by a groundbreaking British Heart study, published in *The Lancet*, in which 7,735 middle-aged men were monitored for more than nine years. The researchers found that the men with the lowest serum albumin levels had the highest rate of death from many different causes, including heart disease. Our levels of serum albumin steadily decline as we age—another indication that albumin may play a role in keeping our bodies healthy, strong, and youthful. Albumin levels are also lower than normal in smokers. Not surprisingly researchers believe that boosting albumin levels will have a salutary effect. They point to test-tube studies confirming that raising albumin levels can both prevent cancerous changes and extend the life span of human cells. Although no such studies have been done on humans, it makes sense that raising albumin levels would help to restore health.

POSSIBLE BENEFITS

Helps cleanse the body of toxins.
Boosts albumin levels.

THE RIGHT AMOUNT

Take up to six 500-mg. tablets daily.

Chondroitin

FACTS

One out of seven Americans will get osteoarthritis, also known as "wear-and-tear" arthritis, which is caused by the wearing down of cartilage, the protective covering that cushions bones. As the cartilage is destroyed, bone rubs against bone, and that can be as uncomfortable as it sounds. Common symptoms of arthritis include stiffness, swelling, and pain in the joints, particularly in the hips and knees. If you complain about arthritic pain, your doctor will probably recommend one of several nonsteroidal anti-inflammatory drugs (NSAIDs) that help reduce the pain but do little to cure the underlying condition that causes the problem: the loss of cartilage. Until recently, it was widely believed that it was impossible to regrow cartilage, but there is compelling new evidence that cartilage can be regenerated. What is even more exciting is the fact that the arthritis "cure" is not some high-tech, expensive medicine concocted by drug companies but a combination of three inexpensive supplements that are sold in natural food stores: chondroitin, glucosamine (page 63), and pregnenolone (see page 131).

Chondroitin, which is found in high concentration in the gristle around the joints of animals, draws fluid to the cells in the joint; that fluid provides lubrication and helps bone glide smoothly with each movement. In addition, chondroitin works with glucosamine to replenish collagen and other components that provide the building blocks for cartilage. Several clinical studies, all performed outside the United States, clearly showed that when arthritic patients were given chondroitin sulfates, they not only experienced significant relief in pain and an increase in mobility but felt positive effects long after they discontinued taking the chondroitin. This is good evidence that the treatment did not simply mask the pain but actually helped to restore lost cartilage.

Several other supplements in the Hot 100 can also help reduce the inflammation and pain typical of arthritis, and they can be used with glucosamine, chondroitin, and pregnenolone. If you are relying on NSAIDs to control your pain, I recommend that you try these natural remedies. Unlike NSAIDs, they do not cause stomach distress or other unpleasant side effects.

POSSIBLE BENEFITS

Reduces arthritic pain.
Regrows cartilage.

THE RIGHT AMOUNT

Take two 500-mg. tablets or capsules twice daily.

Chromium Picolinate

FACTS

Chromium, a mineral I have discussed in earlier books, has recently been "discovered" by fitness buffs and couch potatoes who only want to *look* as if they spend their days working out. Chromium picolinate, the most absorbable form of chromium, is one of the hottest sports supplements around. But before I tell you why the pumping iron set has gone chromium crazy, let me give you some background information.

For years, I have been touting the benefits of chromium picolinate as a natural remedy for elevated blood cholesterol and triglycerides, which can increase the risk of heart attack and stroke. Although chromium lowers the level of "bad" LDL cholesterol, it increases "good" HDL cholesterol, which can protect against heart disease. Chromium picolinate works particularly well in combination with "no-flush" niacin (a special formulation of niacin that avoids gastrointestinal discomfort) to correct these potentially harmful lipid abnormalities. Many physicians also use chromium picolinate to treat Type II diabetes, or insulin resistance, a condition in which the body produces enough insulin but the cells do not use it efficiently, resulting in a rise in blood sugar. About 25 percent of all adults over 40 will develop some form of insulin resistance. Obesity and a diet high in refined sugar increase the likelihood of developing Type II diabetes, but taking chromium picolinate may help prevent or reverse this condition. According to studies performed by the U.S.D.A. Human Nutrition Research Center, chromium can lower blood sugar as effectively as prescription medication, without the side effects.

Dieters and body builders are excited about chromium because of recent studies showing that this mineral can help trim fat and build muscle. In one study conducted at Bemidji State University in Minnesota, one group of male athletes took 200 mcg. daily and another group took a placebo. After six weeks, the men taking chromium gained 44 percent more lean body mass, whereas the gain in the placebo group was only 7 percent. Other studies have shown that it is not necessary to pump iron to gain the benefits of chromium picolinate—you can do nothing and still see some benefits. The effect of chromium supplements on overweight people has been studied. Overweight volunteers at a San Antonio weight loss center were given chromium supplements or a placebo for an average of 72 days and were not given any particular diet or exercise regimen. During the time they were taking chromium, the volunteers lost an average of 4.2 fat pounds and gained 1.4 pounds in lean mass. While they were taking the placebo, however, the changes in body composition were negligible. This meant that chromium picolinate could burn fat and enhance muscle even without exercise or a special diet. Of course, to obtain the full benefits of chromium picolinate, you should follow a sound diet and exercise regularly.

About 90 percent of the population does not get enough chromium from food. (Food sources of chromium include broccoli, brewer's yeast, and shellfish.) To make matters worse, the high-sugar diet typical of many Americans can increase the excretion of chromium, leaving less chromium in the body. Many researchers believe that chromium deficiency may be why Type II diabetes is a virtual epidemic in the United States.

Here's yet another reason to take chromium picolinate: it may help you live longer. A now famous study showed that when rats were fed chromium in their food throughout their lives, they lived 36 percent longer. In human terms, that would be the equivalent of adding 25 years to your life!

POSSIBLE BENEFITS

Burns fat, increases muscle mass.
Reduces cholesterol and triglycerides.
Prevents insulin resistance.

THE RIGHT AMOUNT

Take up to three 200-mcg. capsules daily.

Ciwuja

FACTS

Can an ancient Chinese herb improve athletic performance and endurance? There's exciting new evidence that it can. The root of the ciwuja plant has been used in traditional Chinese medicine for more than 1,700 years to treat fatigue and boost immune function.

Ciwuja attracted the attention of medical researchers who had heard anecdotal reports of its use by mountain climbers to improve performance at high altitudes, where there are low levels of oxygen. Recent studies performed in the United States and China show that ciwuja can indeed improve workout performance, which is why sports supplements containing ciwuja are fast becoming a favorite among fitness mavens. Ciwuja products are also marketed as herbal energizers for anyone who needs an energy boost.

In different studies, researchers at the Academy of Preventive Medicine in Beijing, China, and the Department of Physiology at the University of North Texas Health Science Center discovered that ciwuja can alter normal metabolism during exercise so that more fat and less carbohydrate are burned. This function is beneficial because the shift from carbohydrate to fat burning delays the buildup of lactic acid in the muscles, which can promote fatigue and muscle pain. If you take ciwuja, you can work out longer and harder before feeling tired. The other benefit, of course, is that you will burn more fat.

Even better, ciwuja does not contain steroids or stimulants such as caffeine, and it is safe even at high doses. The growing popularity of supplements such as ciwuja is another example of how savvy athletes are rejecting dangerous drugs in favor of safe, natural supplements that have withstood the test of time.

Ciwuja is often found in supplements that contain other performance-enhancing compounds including Siberian ginseng (see page 184), licorice (see page 192), and bee pollen.

POSSIBLE BENEFITS

Enhances athletic performance.
Increases stamina.

THE RIGHT AMOUNT

Take two 400-mg. capsules daily.

Coenzyme-Q10 (Co-Q10)

FACTS

When I first began writing about supplements more than 20 years ago, Co-Q10 was exotic and hard to find. Today, there are numerous brands of Co-Q10 on the market, and it is now included in many combination formulas promoting weight loss and cardiac health. Co-Q10 is essential for the production of energy in the body, which means that it is essential for life. Co-Q10 helps meet this need for energy by stimulating the mitochondria, the tiny powerhouses within the cells that produce adenosine triphosphate (ATP), the fuel that runs the body. Because Co-Q10 facilitates the production of energy, it may—at least indirectly—help burn calories that would normally be converted to fat. Co-Q10 is best known as a heart-healthy supplement because it is a highly effective treatment for congestive heart failure. In fact, in one study published in the *American Journal of Cardiology*, heart patients taking Co-Q10 either alone or with other drugs lived an average of three years longer than those not taking Co-Q10! Co-Q10 can also lower blood pressure, which can reduce the risk of having a heart attack or stroke.

Perhaps the most intriguing use for Co-Q10 is as a treatment for gum disease, the bane of baby boomers. Researchers at Osaka University in Japan gave patients with gum disease 60 mg. a day of Co-Q10 or a placebo, and no other treatment. After eight weeks, the group taking the Co-Q10 showed marked improvement in their gums, including a reduction in discomfort and inflammation, compared with the placebo group. I have also heard numerous anecdotal accounts of Co-Q10 virtually curing gum disease. If you have mild gum disease, I think it is advisable to try Co-Q10 for two months before submitting to painful, expensive (and often unnecessary) gum treatments. (Of course, if you wait until your mouth is infected and filled with abscesses, you will have no choice but to seek immediate treatment.)

There is a promising new use for Co-Q10. Recently, studies in Europe conducted by Dr. Karl Folkers, who has been researching Co-Q10 for nearly 40 years, have shown that breast cancer patients who took high doses of Co-Q10 daily (over 300 mg. daily) had complete regression of their tumors. I am eagerly awaiting the results of follow-up studies to see whether Co-Q10 can be added to the arsenal of natural cancer fighters.

POSSIBLE BENEFITS

Strengthens the heart.
Lowers high blood pressure.
Reverses gum disease.

THE RIGHT AMOUNT

Take two 60-mg. capsules daily.

Personal Advice

I take a gel form of Co-Q10. It is the best absorbed form, and the capsules are easy to swallow.

Conjugated Linoleic Acid (CLA)

FACTS

It's called the American Paradox. Although dieting is the national pastime, Americans are actually getting *fatter*. In fact, one out of three Americans is obese, which is defined as 30 percent above their ideal body weight. Why? Ironically, some scientists believe that in our quest to lose weight, we are not eating enough fat, or at least the *right* kind of fat. The fat that is missing from our diet is conjugated linoleic acid (CLA), which is found in red meat, lamb, and dairy products. Although these foods contain some of this good fat, they do not get a clean bill of health, since they are very high in calories and are also packed with saturated fat, which can promote cancer and heart disease.

What's good about CLA? It helps the body regulate fat and protein metabolism. Numerous studies have shown that CLA can offer some spectacular health benefits, and in particular can reduce the amount of body fat while increasing muscle. Since muscle burns excess calories, the more muscle you have, the less likely you are to become overweight.

It is very difficult to get enough CLA from food alone. For one thing, many of us avoid foods that are rich in CLA. For another, changes in livestock feeding methods have caused the CLA content in food to decline by nearly 80 percent over the past two decades.

We can make up for this shortfall by taking CLA supplements. Laboratory studies have shown that CLA can block cancer formation in animals exposed to known carcinogens and can also prevent atherosclerosis, or hardening of the arteries. CLA can also raise HDL or "good" cholesterol and can lower elevated triglycerides, a major risk factor for heart disease. It is no surprise that CLA supplements are gaining in popularity. In fact, not only has CLA attracted the attention of people who want to shed excess weight, it is fast becoming a favorite among body builders who want to maximize their muscles.

POSSIBLE BENEFITS

Reduces body fat.
Promotes weight loss.
Enhances muscle tone.
Prevents heart disease.
Protects against many different types of cancer.

THE RIGHT AMOUNT

Take three 600–1200-mg. capsules daily before meals.

Cordyceps (*Cordyceps sinensis*)

FACTS

Cordyceps is an ancient Chinese tonic herb that was traditionally used to fight fatigue and promote vitality. Also known as Chinese caterpillar fungus, cordyceps is actually a parasitic mushroom that grows on certain species of caterpillar. Don't be put off by this unattractive description; real cordyceps is rare and highly prized. In fact, thousands of years ago it was so precious that it was used exclusively in the emperor's palace. In the 1970s, the Chinese government sponsored an all-out project to find ways to cultivate this precious herb cheaply. The scarcity problem was solved a decade later when scientists isolated the active component of cordyceps and created a method of mass-producing it through fermentation.

What's so special about cordyceps? In China, it is considered nothing less than the antidote for old age. Chinese researchers report that older people who take this herb feel stronger and more energetic. In fact, studies have shown that cordyceps can raise levels of naturally produced antioxidants, such as superoxide dismutase, one of the body's primary weapons against free radical damage. The age-related decline in these antioxidants is believed to be a causative factor in many diseases, such as arthritis and heart disease, and even in the aging process itself.

According to Chinese studies, cordyceps can also improve athletic performance. It is widely used by Chinese athletes. Proponents of cordyceps point to the remarkable story of eight Chinese women runners who in 1993 set world records in nearly every competition at their national games in Beijing, the same year they incorporated cordyceps into their diet. Researchers speculate that cordyceps may improve athletic performance by opening up the breathing passages, thereby allowing more oxygen into the body. Oxygen is critical for the production of energy by the cells, and more energy means more endurance. Interestingly, Chinese healers have used cordyceps to treat bronchitis and asthma. In China, cordyceps is also used to restore energy in heart patients who suffer from excessive fatigue.

Athletes and body builders are now using cordyceps in the United States, and it is fast becoming a popular sports supplement. Look for products containing cordyceps combined with other Chinese tonic herbs.

POSSIBLE BENEFITS

Increases stamina.
Protects against free radicals.
Restores energy.

THE RIGHT AMOUNT

Take two 525-mg. capsules daily with meals.

Coriolus Versicolor Extract (PSK)

FACTS

Coriolus versicolor extract is derived from an edible mushroom popular in Asia. In Japan, coriolus versicolor extract is widely used as a government-approved, nontoxic cancer treatment called PSK, or Crestin. It is now available as a nutritional supplement in the United States. For nearly 20 years, researchers have monitored numerous patients taking coriolus, and the results are quite impressive.

In studies where coriolus is used in combination with other cancer treatments, such as radiation, chemotherapy, and surgery, patient survival rates are significantly improved. Although the anticancer properties of coriolus are not fully understood, studies show that it enhances immune function. Notably, coriolus boosts the activity of natural killer cells, which help the body get rid of cancerous growths before they can spread. In test tube studies, it can inhibit the growth of tumors, which suggests it may do the same in humans.

In Japan, coriolus is not touted as a miracle cure; rather, it is an important part of an overall cancer treatment program. In the United States, natural healers are using coriolus versicolor extract for cancer along with other natural therapies, as well as for other diseases related to impaired immune function, including AIDS. Natural healers also report the successful use of coriolus as a treatment for autoimmune problems, such as rheumatoid arthritis and lupus, which occur when immune cells become confused and begin to attack the body's own tissue. Interestingly, although coriolus activates the disease-fighting cells of the immune system, it also has a positive effect on maintaining the right levels of special T-cells called suppressor cells, which prevent the body from attacking itself.

Coriolus is not just for the sick. It may help to maintain immune function in the healthy. In one study, healthy people who were given 1 gram daily experienced a rise in disease-fighting T-cells within 24 hours. As of this writing, coriolus is available only in higher doses (3-gram capsules) for people undergoing medical treatment. It is somewhat expensive compared with other supplements, but it is a veritable bargain in comparison with the cost of many cancer drugs. A lower-dose, relatively inexpensive coriolus product should soon be available. If you are undergoing treatment for cancer or impaired immune function, consult with your physician or natural healer before incorporating coriolus into your treatment.

POSSIBLE BENEFITS

Boosts and normalizes immune function.
Improves effect of other cancer therapies.

THE RIGHT AMOUNT

The usual dose for cancer patients is 3 grams daily. If you are undergoing treatment for cancer or other medical problems, work with a qualified professional.

Creatine Monohydrate

FACTS

Creatine monohydrate is a *superhot* new "sports supplement" that is fast becoming a favorite of body builders and athletes. Creatine is an amino acid that occurs naturally in our bodies and is concentrated in skeletal muscles. It is essential for the production of adenosine triphosphate (ATP), the cellular fuel that runs the body. Creatine is also found in foods such as meat and fish. We consume about 1 gram of creatine daily from our food alone, but for active people, that is not enough.

About 95 percent of the creatine in humans is in skeletal muscle; the rest is in the heart, brain, and testes. Vigorous exercise depletes the muscles of their natural supply of creatine. Creatine supplements help to reenergize tired muscle cells, allowing you to work out harder for a longer time. Several studies, including one recently reported in the *International Journal of Sports Nutrition*, have shown that people who take creatine supplements and exercise regularly lose more fat and develop better muscle tone than people who only work out and do not take creatine supplements. Another study jointly performed by Texas Woman's University, the University of Texas Southwestern Medical Center, and the Cooper Clinic found that creatine enhanced the performance of male weight lifters, allowing them to lift heavier loads and do more repetitions.

Creatine is not necessarily a tool for weight loss, however. In fact, when you gain muscle, you may actually put on a few pounds because muscle weighs more than fat, but you will look slimmer and sleeker.

Although there is no scientific evidence yet to back this claim, I have heard numerous anecdotes from friends and sport trainers who swear that creatine has improved their stamina and increased their strength. Some studies suggest, however, that creatine is not particularly useful for athletes who are engaged in sports that require speed, such as running, where bigger muscles may simply weigh you down.

There is even more good news about creatine: A recent study performed at the Cooper Clinic and Texas Woman's University showed that it can lower elevated levels of total cholesterol and triglycerides, fat-like substances found in the blood. High levels of triglycerides increase the risk of heart disease and stroke.

In Europe, creatine is also being studied as a possible treatment for sarcopenia, the muscle atrophy that can occur as part of the aging process. Starting at about age 30, we may lose an average of 2 to 4 pounds of muscle a decade, and the loss may be accelerated later in life. A sedentary lifestyle is one factor that may trigger muscle loss, and it can be a devastating problem for older people. Creatine may prove to be useful in helping older people maintain their muscles and their strength.

POSSIBLE BENEFITS

Helps to enhance the benefits from your workout.
Builds lean body mass, burns fat.
May protect against heart disease by reducing blood lipid levels.

THE RIGHT AMOUNT

Creatine monohydrate is the form used in supplements because it is most easily absorbed by the body. Creatine is available as a powder, which can be mixed in water or juice, or as chewable wafers. Take 5000 mg. (1 tablespoon of powder) in juice or water daily.

Cryptoxanthin

FACTS

Every time you bite into a peach, papaya, tangerine, or orange, you are getting a healthy serving of cryptoxanthin, one of a select group of carotenoids that can be converted to vitamin A in the body. Two groups of people need to be concerned about getting enough cryptoxanthin: people who smoke or use tobacco products, and women. A 1993 study comparing blood carotenoid levels of women with cervical cancer and cancer-free women found that cancer-free women had significantly higher blood levels of cryptoxanthin, which suggests that cryptoxanthin may offer some protection against this form of cancer. If cryptoxanthin proves to protect against cancer, it would not be the first time that a carotenoid has been shown to have strong anticancer activity. Other studies have revealed that alpha carotene, beta carotene, and lycopene, among others, are potent free radical scavengers and cancer fighters.

Another new study suggests that cryptoxanthin may be depleted by smoking. Scientists compared the blood levels of vitamin E and carotenoids in men who chewed or smoked tobacco with blood levels in those who abstained from tobacco products. Tobacco users had significantly lower levels of cryptoxanthin than those who were tobacco free, which suggests that they should either eat more cryptoxanthin-rich foods or take a carotenoid supplement with cryptoxanthin. (Of course, they should also quit smoking!) Considering that nearly half of all Americans do not eat even one serving of fruit a day, it's a good idea to include this supplement in your daily regimen. Cryptoxanthin is included in mixed carotenoid formulas.

POSSIBLE BENEFITS

May protect against cervical cancer.

THE RIGHT AMOUNT

Take 3 to 6 mg. of mixed carotenoids daily.

Curcumin

FACTS

Curcumin is derived from turmeric, the spice that gives curry powder its distinctive yellow color. (Curcumin is *not* the same as cumin, which may also be found in curry powder.) Turmeric, known as the "spice of life," is widely used in Indian cooking. For thousands of years, turmeric has also been an important part of the Ayurvedic system of medicine practiced by Indian healers. Long before the discovery of refrigeration, curry powders and other spices were used to preserve food, which over time would grow rancid if exposed to oxygen. Not surprisingly, studies have revealed that curcumin is a potent antioxidant.

Today, curcumin is included in many herbal formulas designed to relieve rheumatoid arthritis. Indian studies have shown that curcumin is as strong an anti-inflammatory as many of the arthritis drugs sold by prescription and over the counter. In fact, in double-blind studies with arthritis patients, curcumin produced significant improvement comparable with phenylbutazone, a prescription nonsteroidal anti-inflammatory (NSAID) medication. The advantage of curcumin over the NSAID is that there are no known side effects, while NSAIDs in general can cause stomach distress, bleeding ulcers, and other problems.

Recently, scientists at the American Institute for Cancer Research have begun testing curcumin as a possible treatment for skin, breast, and colon cancer. Earlier, researchers at Pennsylvania State University found that curcumin appears to inhibit the activity of certain proteins that may trigger the growth of breast tumors.

Curcumin also protects against heart disease in several important ways. First, it can lower high blood cholesterol levels, and second, it can prevent blood clots that can lead to heart attack and stroke.

Turmeric, a longtime folk remedy for liver disorders, can reduce inflammation in the liver and strengthen liver function. Today, natural healers often prescribe curcumin to people with hepatitis C, a common liver ailment. To add to its versatility, curcumin has also been used as an effective treatment for gallbladder disease.

POSSIBLE BENEFITS

Reduces inflammation from rheumatoid arthritis.

Antioxidant action may help protect against cancer and heart disease.

THE RIGHT AMOUNT

Take up to three 500-mg. capsules daily with food. Look for 18:1 concentration.

Personal Advice

If you smoke, please quit as soon as possible. But until you do, be sure to add curcumin to your supplement regimen. One fascinating study showed that high doses of curcumin could reduce the free radical damage inflicted on smokers by the hundreds of carcinogenic chemicals in cigarettes. I'm not saying that turmeric can help prevent smoking-related ailments, only that it may postpone some of the damage.

Cynarin (Artichoke Concentrate)

FACTS

A compound found in artichokes, cynarin has been used in Europe for several decades to lower elevated blood lipids (such as high cholesterol and triglycerides) which can greatly increase the risk of heart disease. More than 50 years ago, Japanese researchers found that artichokes can boost the production of bile by the liver, which in turn is used to break down fat. Cholesterol-lowering drugs can in rare cases cause liver damage, but cynarin is actually beneficial for liver function. In fact, cynarin is a close botanical cousin of the herb milk thistle, which is well known for its positive effect on liver health.

Studies have shown that cynarin can reduce elevated triglycerides, lower total serum cholesterol, and raise levels of beneficial, or good, HDL. While many people watch their cholesterol levels, they may be unaware that a high triglyceride level (over 200 mg./dl. for women and 400 mg./dl. for men) is a serious risk factor for heart disease and stroke, especially for women. In fact, according to the famous Framingham study, a high triglyceride level in postmenopausal women is as important a risk factor for heart disease as high cholesterol.

If you have moderately high blood cholesterol or triglycerides, try using natural products such as cynarin to bring them down to normal levels.

POSSIBLE BENEFITS

May prevent heart disease by lowering blood lipid levels. Enhances liver function.

THE RIGHT AMOUNT

Take four 500-mg. capsules daily. You should see an improvement in blood lipid levels within two months.

Deglycyrrhizinated Licorice (DGL)

FACTS

Check out the natural food stores for DGL, a new form of licorice, a traditional favorite herb. Among Asian healers, licorice is highly regarded as a treatment for ulcers, arthritis, and even cancer. Two thousand years ago, it was one of a select group of herbs listed in the renowned Chinese *Shennong Herbal*. We have long known that licorice contains a natural anti-inflammatory agent that not only is good for arthritis-type joint pain but can relieve gastrointestinal symptoms due to ulcers. As effective as licorice may be for treating these problems, many people were advised to avoid it because it can raise blood pressure. The good news is that DGL does not contain glycyrrhetinic acid, the compound in licorice that can raise blood pressure. Yet, it still offers many of the same benefits of licorice, especially when it comes to soothing gastrointestinal problems.

If you frequently use antacids for heartburn or ulcer pain, you should know that DGL is superior to over-the-counter and prescription antacids in several ways. Antacids work by reducing acid secretions in the stomach, which can interrupt normal digestion and may cause problems later. In fact, it is very common for people with excess acid or ulcer pain to have frequent recurrences. However, DGL works by increasing the protective lining in the stomach and small intestine, providing a natural buffer against stomach acid, and this may actually help to prevent future problems. Several clinical studies, including one in the prestigious British medical journal *The Lancet*, concluded that DGL worked better than many popular prescription treatments for duodenal ulcers. In fact, patients taking DGL healed faster and had fewer relapses than those using other drugs. And unlike prescription or over-the-counter antacids, DGL does not cause unwanted side effects such as nausea, diarrhea, or possible liver damage. Even better, it is much less expensive than many other medications.

POSSIBLE BENEFITS

Relieves pain due to ulcers or excess gas.
Helps reduce pain from arthritis.

THE RIGHT AMOUNT

For gastrointestinal pain, chew two 380-mg. tablets 20 minutes before eating.

Decosahexaenoic Acid (DHA)

FACTS

If you're like most people, you've probably spent the last decade counting your fat grams because of studies that linked a high-fat diet to an increased risk of heart disease and cancer. But in your zeal to eat right, you may have eliminated some good fats in the process, notably decosahexaenoic acid (DHA), an essential fatty acid that cannot be manufactured by the body. DHA is found in foods that many people have given up in the name of good health, such as organ meats (which are high in both saturated fat and toxins) and eggs (which may be too high in cholesterol for people with lipid problems). It is also abundant in fatty fish, like salmon, mackerel, sardines, and albacore tuna; however, most Americans do not eat significant quantities of fish. Why do we need DHA? DHA is found in high concentration in the gray matter of the brain and the retina of the eye. It is also instrumental in the function of brain cell membranes, which are important for the transmission of brain signals.

Essential for normal brain and eye development, DHA is passed from the mother to the fetus via the placenta. After birth, the primary source of DHA is breast milk. Over the past 50 years, the consumption of DHA has significantly declined, and this has many scientists worried. According to an article published in the *American*

Journal of Clinical Nutrition, Dr. Joseph R. Hibbeln and Dr. Norman Salem of the National Institutes of Health linked the increase in depression in North America over the past century to a steady decline in DHA consumption. The authors noted that in countries where DHA consumption has remained high, depression is not as common. Low levels of DHA have also been associated with an increase in dementia, mood changes, memory loss, and visual problems. In fact, in a Swedish study, elderly patients with Alzheimer's disease were found to have lower blood levels of DHA than healthy older people. Another Japanese study showed a 65 percent improvement in dementia symptoms among patients given DHA supplements.

Scientists are also concerned about the decline of DHA in breast milk, and they fear that it may interfere with normal mental development in children. In Europe, DHA is added to infant formulas. Although there is no direct evidence that links DHA to mental or behavior problems in children, at least one study performed at Purdue University found that boys diagnosed with attention deficit hyperactivity disorder had lower levels of essential fatty acids, such as DHA, in their blood than children who did not have this problem. In addition, some scientists speculate that the deficiency of DHA may be a contributing factor in postpartum depression in new mothers.

POSSIBLE BENEFITS

May prevent depression.
Can reduce symptoms of dementia.
Promotes normal brain development in children.
Enhances vision.

THE RIGHT AMOUNT

Take up to three 250-mg. capsules daily.

Personal Advice

If you are a nursing mother, check with your physician or natural healer about taking DHA. It may be just what you and your baby need to be happier and healthier!

Dehydroepiandrosterone (DHEA)

FACTS

You've undoubtedly seen the signs in the natural food stores proclaiming "We have DHEA," and you may have wondered what the fuss was all about. In a word, it's about health and about our ability to maintain our health throughout old age.

Dehydroepiandrosterone (DHEA) is a natural hormone that is produced in the brain, skin, and adrenal glands. It is the most abundant steroid hormone in the body. As we age our levels of DHEA drop, so that about the age of 45, we produce only *half* of the DHEA we produced at age 20. Many scientists believe that the decline in key hormones such as DHEA is responsible for much of the physical and mental decline we have come to associate with normal aging. Therefore, they believe that by boosting DHEA back to youthful levels, we may be able to prevent and even reverse some of these problems.

I have been taking DHEA for the past two years, and I have found that it has a wonderful effect on my energy levels. I live an extraordinarily active life: writing, traveling, lecturing, and spending time with my family. Since I have been taking DHEA, I find that I have more stamina and am better able to maintain my rigorous schedule. I have heard dozens of stories similar to mine, and I truly believe that this hormone has an energizing effect on the body.

Hundreds of studies have documented the vital role that DHEA plays in the body, but it appears to be especially important for normal immune function. As we get older our immune system weakens, making us more vulnerable to infection, cancer, and even autoimmune diseases such as rheumatoid arthritis. There is good evidence that DHEA supplementation can *reverse* many of the problems that arise in immune function as we age. In a recent study conducted by Dr. Omid Khorram, a professor of medicine at the University of San Diego, nine healthy older men were given DHEA supplements for five months. Dr. Khorram found that DHEA stimulated the production of immune cells that fight against viruses and bacteria, as well as important cells called natural killer cells, which help weed out cancerous cells before they can grow.

In addition to boosting immune function, DHEA appears to have a significant effect on our emotional well-being. In a recent study conducted at the University of San Diego, DHEA supplements were given to 13 men and 17 women, aged 40 to 70, for three months. For another three months, the group received a placebo. During the time they were taking the DHEA, the researchers reported a "remarkable increase in perceived physical and psychological well-being for both men and women." The men and women not only felt better when they were taking DHEA but said they were better able to cope with stress.

Other studies have shown that low levels of DHEA increase the risk of heart disease in men. And interestingly, in one study of men over the age of 40, low levels of DHEA were strongly correlated with sexual dysfunction.

Even though DHEA is sold over the counter, it is still wise to have your DHEA levels checked by your doctor so you can see whether you need this supplement. DHEA is not necessary for most people under 40, whose bodies are probably making enough of it. People in their mid-40s and beyond will probably find that they are low in DHEA.

Recently, researchers at Stanford University Medical Center tested DHEA in women with lupus, a potentially debilitating autoimmune disorder that is marked by joint pain, skin rashes, excess fatigue, chest pain, and a susceptibility to infection. In serious cases, lupus can lead to kidney disease. There is no cure for lupus, and the drug therapies, ranging from prednisone to NSAIDs to antimalarials to strong chemotherapy drugs, can all cause serious side effects. In two small studies, researchers gave lupus patients 200 mg. of DHEA daily for up to three months. The results were very encouraging. In fact, not only did most of the patients feel markedly better, but their blood tests showed less autoimmune activity. Even better, there were minimal side effects. Anyone with lupus should certainly talk to his or her physician about trying DHEA.

POSSIBLE BENEFITS

Strengthens the immune system.
Enhances mood.
May reduce symptoms of autoimmune diseases such as lupus and rheumatoid arthritis.

THE RIGHT AMOUNT

The usual dose is one 50-mg. tablet daily for men over age 40, and one 25-mg. tablet daily for women over age 40. For best results, take DHEA in the morning.

CAUTION

If you have a history of prostate cancer or breast cancer, I advise that you not use DHEA. Although there is absolutely no evidence that DHEA is harmful, it is a hormone and can theoretically stimulate the growth of hormone-dependent cancers.

Personal Advice

Look for "pharmaceutical grade" on the DHEA label—it ensures as pure a product as possible.

Elderberry Extract (*Sambucus nigra*)

FACTS

When Israeli pilots feel a cold or flu coming on, they reach for Sambucol, a brand of Israeli elderberry extract that is gaining popularity throughout the world. They are grounded until they are better, but within a day or two they are typically back in action. Since the days of Hippocrates, elderberry has been reputed to be the best herbal therapy for fevers and colds, but it was only very recently that researchers at Hadassah University Medical Center in Jerusalem unraveled the science behind the folk cure.

In 1992, a team of Israeli scientists and physicians conducted a double-blind study testing elderberry extract on 50 patients infected with flu virus. Half were given elderberry extract and the other half were given a placebo. Within 24 hours, 20 percent of the elderberry takers showed dramatic improvement in fever, muscle pain, and respiratory symptoms. Amazingly, by the second day, 75 percent showed a real change for the better, and by the third day, 90 percent felt markedly better. Contrast this to the placebo group, in which only 8 percent showed any improvement within 24 hours and 16 percent in 48 hours; the rest took an entire six days to improve.

How does elderberry extract work? A flu virus enters a cell by puncturing the cell membrane (which encases the cell) with tiny spikes covered with an enzyme designed to destroy the cell membrane. Elderberry is rich in bioflavonoids, substances that can strengthen cell membranes and make them less easy to penetrate. In addition, researchers believe that elderberry may inhibit the enzyme that weakens the cell membranes.

Elderberry extract has been tested on a wide variety of flu viruses and is effective against all of them. In addition, preliminary test tube studies suggest that elderberry can inhibit the AIDS virus, but more studies need to be done to see if it works as well in humans.

POSSIBLE BENEFITS

Can relieve symptoms of cold and flu.

THE RIGHT AMOUNT

At the first sign of a cold or flu, take two 500-mg. capsules daily, or take one tablespoon of elderberry extract every four hours for up to four days.

Emu Oil

FACTS

Several of the Hot 100 supplements come to us from remote parts of the world where they have been used in traditional medicine. One of the more intriguing of these newly discovered supplements is an oil derived from the fat of the emu, a bird that is native to Australia and a close relative of the ostrich. Australian doctors learned about emu oil from native Aboriginal tribesmen, who have long used it as a sunscreen and to treat skin wounds and joint pain.

Products made from emu oil—ranging from soothing balms for arthritis to antiaging skin creams—are sold in pharmacies and department stores throughout Australia and are now appearing on the shelves of natural food stores in the United States.

Emu oil is a rich source of linolenic acid, which can reduce the swelling, stiffness and inflammation typical of arthritis. Although large clinical studies on arthritis and emu oil have not yet been conducted, there is a wealth of anecdotal evidence attesting to its effectiveness. The rediscovery of emu oil by modern medicine is being credited to Dr. Peter Ghosh, director of the research lab at Sydney's Royal North Shore Hospital and a leading authority on arthritis. On the basis of small studies involving his patients, Dr. Ghosh reports that emu oil offers the "best relief ever" for arthritis.

Major burn centers worldwide are reporting that emu oil, long used by Aboriginal healers to treat wounds and burns, can help promote healing. An excellent moisturizer for the skin, emu oil is reputed to reduce fine lines and wrinkles and to protect against sun damage. In Australia, emu oil is recommended as a treatment for sunburn.

I recently learned of one breast cancer patient, undergoing radiation therapy, who used emu oil successfully to protect her skin against radiation burns. According to this report, she suffered little pain and healed faster than other patients.

Emus are farm-raised birds; every part of the emu is used. Emu meat, which is popular in Australia, looks and tastes like beef but is as low in fat and cholesterol as turkey meat.

POSSIBLE BENEFITS

Relieves arthritic symptoms.
Promotes wound healing.
Soothes muscle aches and sprains.

THE RIGHT AMOUNT

For joint or muscle pain, massage into affected areas two or three times daily. For burns and wounds, use as directed.

Personal Advice

Try using emu oil to reduce post-workout soreness and muscle strains.

Flaxseed Oil

FACTS

It seems that everyone from the scientists at the National Cancer Institute to natural healers is singing the praises of flaxseed oil, which is why it earns a spot on my elite Hot 100. Like so many "new" supplements, flaxseed oil reminds us yet again that there is nothing new under the sun. About 8,500 years ago, our hunter/gatherer ancestors ate flax along with other wild grasses. Every part of the plant was put to good use. The oil from the seeds was used for cooking and making paint; the plant fiber was spun into rope and cloth. The flax plant is still used to make cloth, paper, and other products, but only recently have there been serious attempts to reintroduce it into our modern diet.

Flaxseed is one of the best sources of omega-3 fatty acids, a type of "good" fat that is missing from the typical Western diet. Scientists at the National Cancer Institute became interested in omega-3 fatty acids in general, and flaxseed oil in particular, after numerous European studies had shown that omega-3 fatty acids can shrink cancerous tumors and have a potent anticancer effect on breast, prostate, and lung cancer cells.

In addition to containing omega-3 fatty acids, flaxseed oil is a rich source of lignans, a type of fiber that is changed by "friendly bacteria" in the gut into compounds that fight against cancer. Lignans can also modulate hormone levels and relieve some of the symptoms often associated with menopause, such as hot flashes and yeast infections due to vaginal dryness. Flaxseed oil is also a treatment for premenstrual syndrome, which may be caused by a hormonal imbalance.

To add to their many benefits, omega-3 fatty acids contain a natural anti-inflammatory agent that can help relieve the symptoms of rheumatoid arthritis, psoriasis, allergies, and other inflammatory diseases. Natural healers routinely prescribe flaxseed oil for these conditions, often with great success.

In addition to protecting against cancer, omega-3 fatty acids offer important protection against heart disease, as has been shown by hundreds of studies. Omega-3 fatty acids can lower high cholesterol and high blood pressure, reduce elevated blood triglyceride levels, and prevent blood clots. There's yet more good news about omega-3 rich flaxseed oil. Recently, it has been discovered that omega-3 fatty acids can lower blood levels of the protein homocysteine. Elevated levels of homocysteine are believed to be a major risk factor for heart disease.

Body builders claim that flaxseed oil supplements can increase their stamina and help them recover more quickly from workouts. Flaxseed contains a natural antioxidant, which could explain why it helps tired muscles recover more quickly. In addition, its anti-inflammatory effect can also help reduce muscle soreness.

The downside is that flaxseed oil is not easy to use. It is notoriously unstable and, unless it is properly processed, can turn rancid very quickly. Taking flaxseed oil capsules daily is a convenient way to get the full benefits of flaxseed oil without the bother.

POSSIBLE BENEFITS

May help block the growth of cancerous tumors.

Reduces inflammation.

Corrects lipid abnormalities that could increase the risk of heart disease.

Helps to normalize hormone levels.

THE RIGHT AMOUNT

Take three 1000-mg. capsules daily with meals.

Forskolin

FACTS

Forskolin is an extract derived from the *Coleus forsholi* herb, used in the Indian Ayurvedic system of medicine. For centuries, *Coleus forsholi* has been used as a natural remedy for heart disease, psoriasis, and insomnia. Forskolin has been the subject of thousands of studies, primarily conducted in India. Today, Indian physicians use forskolin to treat high blood pressure, angina, and heart failure, when the heart muscle is so weak it cannot pump blood properly.

Studies have shown that forskolin not only can lower both systolic and diastolic blood pressure but also can strengthen the action of the heart muscle, thereby improving blood flow throughout the body. Many alternative physicians in the United States are prescribing forskolin along with other natural remedies for high blood pressure, instead of prescription antihypertensive medications. Although these drugs work well, they often can cause unpleasant side effects, including fatigue, dry mouth, depression, and even impotence. If you are taking medication to lower your blood pressure and want to try forskolin, do not do so on your own. Work with your physician or natural healer to switch slowly from prescription drugs to natural alternatives.

According to animal studies, forskolin may also help prevent glaucoma, one of the leading causes of blindness among the elderly. Glaucoma is caused by a rise in fluid pressure within the eyeball, which can damage the optic nerve. When applied directly on the eye, forskolin reduces intraocular pressure and increases blood flow, which could help prevent and possibly reverse some of the damage inflicted by glaucoma. Forskolin is not yet available in eye drops, but it may have a similar effect if taken orally.

Recently, forskolin has been investigated as a possible anticancer drug. Forskolin has been shown to inhibit the growth of tumors in animals injected with cancerous cells, and it appears to stimulate immune system activity.

Forskolin is good medicine, but it can also be strong medicine. Use this herb as you need it under the direction of a knowledgeable physician or natural healer.

POSSIBLE BENEFITS

Lowers high blood pressure.
Strengthens the heart.
May prevent glaucoma.

THE RIGHT AMOUNT

Forskolin is available in standardized extract and capsules.
Talk to your physician or natural healer to determine the
right dose for you.

CAUTION

If you are taking any prescription medication (antidepressants, antihistamines, etc.) check with your physician before using forskolin.

Fructo-oligosaccharide (FOS)

FACTS

Fructo-oligosaccharide (FOS), a complex sugar derived from plants, is widely used in Japan in more than 450 different food products. Unlike the refined sugar that is popular in the United States, FOS is actually *good* for you. In fact, it offers so many health benefits that it is now being marketed as a nutritional supplement in this country. Also known as neosugar or inulin, FOS is abundant in Jerusalem artichokes and is found in smaller amounts in many different fruits and vegetables. What is unique about FOS is that it is not broken down by digestive juices, like other sugars. Rather, it passes directly to the gut, where it is digested by "good" bacteria, thereby encouraging their growth.

The human body is host to billions of microorganisms—some good, some bad. The good bacteria perform many essential tasks: They aid in digestion, enhance immune function, control the growth of bad bacteria and fungi, and help prevent cancer by maintaining the right acidity levels in the gastrointestinal tract. There are more than 400 different species of bacteria in the gut, but the ones that are most beneficial include *Bifidobacterium bifidum*, *Lactobacillus acidophilus*, and *Lactobacillus bulgaricus*. (For more information, see "Probiotics" on page 135.) Bifidobacteria are particularly important because they are involved in the breakdown of key B vitamins.

To maintain optimum health, it is essential to maintain the right balance between the good and the bad bacteria. Unfortunately, the typical American diet is not conducive to growing good bacteria. Refined sugar, meat, and highly processed foods tip the scales against friendly bacteria and encourage the growth of bad bacteria. If the balance tips too much in favor of bad bacteria, we are at greater risk of developing yeast infections, gastric disorders, and even the formation of carcinogens in the liver and colon, which can lead to cancer. As we age, levels of good bacteria decline, which may be responsible for our greater susceptibility to disease in later years. Studies have shown that when older people are given FOS supplements, their *Bifidobacterium* count increases. There is also a decrease in the pH of the lower intestine, making it inhospitable to bad bacteria.

Japanese studies have shown that eating 3 to 6 grams daily of FOS can reduce the level of toxic cancer-causing compounds in human feces by over 40 percent within three weeks.

What is truly remarkable is that FOS can also *normalize* blood sugar levels. Eating too much refined sugar may cause abnormalities in blood sugar that can lead to problems such as Type II diabetes or insulin resistance. But FOS, according to some studies, can reduce high blood sugar levels in diabetic people and also lower elevated cholesterol levels.

POSSIBLE BENEFITS

Increases levels of good bacteria in the gut.
Enhances immune function.
Lowers elevated blood sugar and cholesterol levels.
Protects against gastrointestinal cancers.

THE RIGHT AMOUNT

FOS is available in powder, which can be mixed in liquid, and capsules. Start with 1 gram daily. If you have chronic Candida albicans (yeast) infection, gas, bloating, or other gastrointestinal problems, you can increase your dose to 4 grams daily.

Personal Advice

Try FOS if you have diarrhea or constipation. It can be taken with other probiotics. Look for food products containing FOS.

Germanium

FACTS

Germanium is a trace element that occurs naturally in food and herbs, such as garlic, shiitake mushroom, ginseng, suma (the South American tonic herb), and aloe vera. In the 1980s, organic germanium (also known as GE 132) became popular after the publication of the book *Miracle Cure: Organic Germanium* by Japanese engineer Kazuhiko

Asai, founder of the Asai Germanium Research Institute. Inorganic germanium was primarily used in industry, but Dr. Asai noticed that many of the most important Chinese herbs contained high amounts of organic germanium, which is safe for human use. In his book, Dr. Asai touted germanium as a nontoxic but potent anticancer treatment, useful for numerous other medical conditions, including rheumatoid arthritis, *Candida albicans* (yeast) infections, and viral infections. After a brief period of intense publicity, germanium fell out of the spotlight.

Recently, organic germanium has been rediscovered because of new studies confirming that it can enhance immune function, particularly in people with autoimmune diseases, in which immune cells attack the body's own tissue. Specifically, organic germanium can stimulate natural killer cells, which weed out cancerous cells and viruses, and can also enhance the activity of disease-fighting T-cells and B-cells. In particular, organic germanium can correct deficiencies in the immune system that lead to autoimmune diseases such as rheumatoid arthritis. Other studies report that germanium can block the growth of many different types of cancers in experimental animals. According to anecdotal reports, organic germanium can also relieve acute pain in cancer patients.

Natural healers and doctors on the cutting edge of alternative medicine use organic germanium to treat the Epstein-Barr virus and other infections that are resistant to antibiotics. This is part of an overall trend to treat disease by strengthening the immune system so that the body can fight its own battles.

POSSIBLE BENEFITS

Enhances immune function.
May protect against cancer.

THE RIGHT AMOUNT

For an active infection, the usual dose is between 50 and 150 mg. daily.

Glucosamine

FACTS

One in five Americans suffers from arthritis, a general term for a problem that encompasses more than 200 different conditions. The most common forms of arthritis are osteoarthritis, also known as wear-and-tear arthritis, and rheumatoid arthritis, caused by inflammation of the joints. Although the two conditions are very different, they are both characterized by the destruction of connective tissue, specifically the cartilage, the substance that lines the joints. When the cartilage wears down, it leaves the bone endings exposed; the result can be pain, stiffness, and swelling of the joints. Recently touted as the so-called arthritis cure, glucosamine is a natural constituent of cartilage that stimulates the production of connective tissue in the body. Although I myself don't feel comfortable calling glucosamine a "cure" for arthritis, I do believe that it can greatly relieve the symptoms associated with this potentially debilitating disorder and can even reverse some of the damage.

As people age they are unable to make enough glucosamine. As a result, the cartilage is unable to retain water and act as a shock absorber. Several studies have shown that glucosamine supplements not only relieve the pain of arthritis but can even halt the progress of the disease. Gradually, over time, glucosamine tackles the underlying cause of arthritis by restoring lost cartilage.

Although anti-inflammatory drugs work faster than glucosamine, glucosamine is more effective over time, primarily because the effect of anti-inflammatory medications can quickly wear off, whereas glucosamine continues to work. Better yet, glucosamine is safe, and there are virtually no side effects. Glucosamine works best with two other supplements, chondroitin (see page 27), which is also found in cartilage, and pregnenolone (see page 131), a natural hormone. This combination not only can reduce the pain of arthritis but will stimulate the production of new cartilage.

POSSIBLE BENEFITS

Relieves and reverses symptoms of arthritis.

THE RIGHT AMOUNT

I recommend glucosamine HCl, which is 40 percent more potent than regular glucosamine. Take up to three 500-mg. tablets daily. I also recommend taking 10 mg. of pregnenolone up to three times daily for maximum relief.

Personal Advice

In rare instances, glucosamine may cause nausea or heartburn. However, this can usually be alleviated by taking it with meals.

L-Glutamine

FACTS

L-glutamine—the natural form of the amino acid glutamine—is amazingly versatile. It is critical for normal brain and immune function, has been used for the treatment of fatigue and alcoholism, and is even reputed to help reduce sugar cravings in people trying to lose weight. Paradoxically, this supplement is primarily used by the very fit and the very sick, for the same reasons: L-glutamine can help build muscle.

L-glutamine is synthesized from three other amino acids: arginine (see page 3), ornithine, and proline. L-glutamine is also a component of glutathione, the body's primary antioxidant, which is present in virtually every cell. If you are deficient in L-glutamine, you are likely to be deficient in glutathione. What is fascinating about glutamine is that it is one of a handful of substances that can naturally boost the level of human growth hormone, which is essential for normal growth and development. Recently, growth hormone has been used experimentally as a treatment for the loss of muscle that often occurs among the sick and the elderly and can lead to wasting syndrome. Although growth hormone can help maintain strength, the problem is that synthetic growth hormone is extremely expensive and can cause unpleasant side effects, such as fluid retention and arthritic symptoms. However, growth hormone–releasing agents, such as glutamine, may offer some of the positive effects of growth hormone, minus the expense or the array of side effects. This is particularly important for people who are severely ill and who often succumb to wasting syndrome. In fact, glutamine is often given to patients with burn injuries to promote healing and to help strengthen immune function. Glutamine has also been used successfully on cancer patients undergoing bone marrow transplant, shortening their stay in the hospital and reducing their risk of infection.

Because of its reputation as a protein-sparing agent, L-glutamine has attracted the attention of fitness buffs who want to lose fat but maintain muscle. People who work out vigorously are at risk of overtaxing their bodies and of losing lean tissue along with the fat. Any supplement that can promote muscle growth will be a hit among the muscle-flexing set, and in fact, L-glutamine is a common ingredient in many sports supplements, including meal replacement powders.

POSSIBLE BENEFITS

Can promote wound healing.
May prevent muscle wasting in the chronically ill.
Enhances muscle size in healthy people who work out.

THE RIGHT AMOUNT

Take up to three 500-mg. capsules or tablets either half an hour before meals or two hours after eating.

Glycerol

FACTS

Unlike the typical sports supplement designed to improve stamina and athletic performance, glycerol is unique: its primary role is to replace the fluid that is lost during exertion. During a strenuous workout you can lose as much as 3 to 4 pounds of fluid, and the loss can be even greater if you are exercising in a warm, humid climate. If the fluid is not replaced, you will not only slow down but run the risk of heat exhaustion and heat stroke. Dehydration results in a reduction in blood plasma, which leaves less blood to carry vital nutrients and oxygen to muscle cells. As a result, you will tire sooner and take longer to recover from your workout. In addition, there is less blood to cool down the skin. Drinking extra water helps to replace fluid, but it may not be enough.

Glycerol is a hydroscopic compound that naturally occurs in every cell of the body and helps cells hold onto water. Glycerol can travel in and out of cells, delivering water where it is needed. Studies have shown that when athletes drink a beverage containing glycerol during strenuous exercise, they lose less fluid and maintain lower body temperatures and a lower heart rate than when they drink water alone. Drinking a glycerol beverage after exercise can help rehydrate the body more quickly. Sports supplements containing glycerol are available at sporting goods stores and natural food stores.

POSSIBLE BENEFITS

Prevents dehydration during exercise.

THE RIGHT AMOUNT

Drink a glycerol sports drink 30 minutes before strenuous exercise, and immediately following exercise. Be sure to drink plenty of water while you exercise. If you are exercising for a long period of time—for example, running a marathon—you may need to replenish glycerol during the race.

Grapefruit Seed Extract

FACTS

Grapefruit seed extract (not to be confused with *grapeseed* extract) is yet one more weapon in the natural arsenal against *Candida albicans*, or yeast infections. *Candida albicans* is one of many different kinds of microorganisms that live within our bodies. Under normal conditions, *Candida albicans* is kept in check by good bacteria that aid in digestion. However, our natural system of checks and balances can become weakened for several reasons. First and foremost is the overuse of antibiotics, which indiscriminately kill both good and bad bacteria, thereby allowing *Candida albicans* to grow out of control. Second, since *Candida albicans* thrives on sugar, the high sugar content typical of the Western diet contributes to this problem.

As a result, recurrent vaginal yeast infections plague many women. In addition, anyone with a weakened immune system is vulnerable to yeast-related ailments, such as thrush or skin rashes. To compound the problem, *Candida albicans* is particularly difficult to defeat because it is very persistent and can quickly grow resistant to treatment. Unfortunately, the over-the-counter treatments are often ineffective—they may work for a short while, but the infection returns.

One way to tackle yeast infections is to increase the level of good bacteria in the gut that helps to keep *Candida albicans* growth under control. (See Probiotics, page 135.) Another way to tip the odds in your favor is to take herbs and other supplements, such as grapefruit seed extract, that have antifungal properties. Although scientific studies are scarce, there is a wealth of anecdotal reports on the use of grapefruit seed extract as a treatment for fungal infections. Grapefruit seed extract contains beneficial bioflavonoids, including hesperidin, which is a natural immune booster. Natural healers report that taken internally, it can help relieve the symptoms of fungal infections for many people.

POSSIBLE BENEFITS

Fights against yeast infections.

THE RIGHT AMOUNT

For internal use, take 10 to 15 drops of grapefruit seed extract in juice or water two to three times daily.

Personal Advice

Grapefruit seed extract can also be used directly on toenail fungus, which is extremely difficult to treat. For external use, rub a few drops of grapefruit seed extract directly on the affected area twice daily until symptoms disappear.

Green-Lipped Mussel Extract

FACTS

New Zealand green-lipped mussel extract is one of three Hot 100 supplements that are derived from marine plants or animals. (The other two are sea cucumber [see page 155] and shark liver oil [see page 157].)

It's ironic that in many ways, we know more about outer space than we do about life beneath our oceans on earth, which are still mostly unexplored. Like the world's rainforests, which contain thousands of species of plants that we have not yet identified, the ocean floor is filled with numerous mysterious plants and creatures that may offer important cures for common diseases. For example, researchers recently have discovered that the green-lipped mussel contains a natural anti-inflammatory agent that is a wonderful treatment for arthritis. Laboratory studies show that green-lipped mussel extract can inhibit the activation of enzymes and other substances that promote inflammation and contribute to the swelling and joint pain typical of arthritis.

When put to the test in arthritis patients, green-lipped mussel extract produced excellent results. In one study conducted at the Glasgow Homeopathic Hospital in Glasgow, Scotland, 66 patients with arthritis were given three 350-mg. capsules of green-lipped mussel extract daily. All of them had such severe arthritic symptoms that they were candidates for joint replacement surgery, and all had been taking nonsteroidal anti-inflammatory drugs (NSAIDs). Despite the severity of the patients' symptoms, researchers reported that 68 percent of those with rheumatoid arthritis and 39.5 percent of those with osteoarthritis showed significant improvement after taking green-lipped mussel extract. The researchers concluded that the treatment "reduces the amount of pain and stiffness, improves the patient's general ability to cope with life, and apparently enhances general health." In addition, unlike NSAIDs, which can cause stomach bleeding and ulcers, green-lipped mussel extract appears to have a gastroprotective effect.

POSSIBLE BENEFITS

Reduces arthritic symptoms.

THE RIGHT AMOUNT

Take three 350-mg. capsules daily for two months. If symptoms abate, try reducing your dose to two 350-mg. capsules. There are no known side effects.

Green Tea Extract

FACTS

Green tea, also known as Chinese tea, has been a popular beverage in Asia for over 3,000 years. Unlike the black tea favored in the West, green tea is more lightly processed and has a distinctively different, delicate flavor. Green tea is not only a satisfying beverage but a rich source of polyphenols—compounds that show great promise as potent cancer fighters. People who regularly drink green tea have lower rates of stomach, lung, esophageal, pancreatic, and colon cancer than those who don't. A particularly interesting study showed that even people who smoked but drank green tea had significantly lower cancer rates than those who smoked but didn't drink green tea. These findings are strengthened by animal studies showing that green tea polyphenols can stimulate the production of important antioxidants and detoxifying enzymes in the body that block cancerous changes. In a study conducted by the American Health Foundation in Valhalla, New York, mice were exposed to strong cancer-causing agents that target lung tissue. Half of the exposed mice were given green tea in their drinking water; the other half were not. Several weeks later, at the study's completion, there were about 45 percent fewer cases of lung cancer among the tea-drinking mice than among the others.

Some studies have even shown green tea polyphenols to have a stronger antioxidant action than vitamins C and E, two of the most powerful antioxidants. In addition, when applied to the skin of animals, green tea polyphenols can prevent skin tumors from forming after exposure to known carcinogens and excessive sunlight. Not surprisingly, skin creams containing green tea polyphenols are now being sold at natural food stores and are being touted as the antidote to sun-damaged skin.

In countries where green tea is routinely consumed, there are also significantly lower levels of heart disease, possibly because of green tea's heart-healthy properties.

Green tea can prevent abnormal blood clotting, lower high blood pressure, lower high cholesterol, and raise the levels of good HDL cholesterol.

To get the full anticancer beneficial effects of green tea, most experts agree that you need to drink between 5 to 10 cups daily, which is unrealistic. Although green tea contains only half the caffeine of coffee, 5 to 10 cups is enough to make you very jittery. (There are some decaffeinated brands, but they are hard to find.) Most brands of green tea tablets are caffeine-free, and many people prefer the convenience.

POSSIBLE BENEFITS

Inhibits formation of cancerous tumors.

Can heal sun-damaged skin.

May prevent many different types of cancers through antioxidant action.

THE RIGHT AMOUNT

I take a combination tablet of green tea extract (no caffeine) and grapeseed extract twice daily. One green tea extract tablet is equal to 1½ cups of green tea.

Personal Advice

When sipped as a beverage, green tea prevents bacteria from sticking to teeth, thus preventing cavities. If you don't drink tea, you can open one capsule into a cup of warm water and simply wash your mouth with the contents.

If you have a sunburn, gently pat some cool green tea on the burned area to relieve the pain and promote healing.

Guarana

FACTS

Grown in the wild Amazon region of Brazil and Uruguay, the fruit of the guarana plant is one of the most popular herbs in the southern hemisphere. In fact, in South America, guarana is synonymous with energy. Guarana is considered a tonic herb; that is, unlike some herbs that are used for their medicinal properties, guarana is primarily used as a general revitalizer. Throughout South America, guarana is widely used in beverages, cereals, and candy. It is now available in capsules at natural food stores in the United States.

Guarana contains caffeine, a natural stimulant also found in coffee, tea, and cola drinks. Each 500-mg. capsule of guarana contains about 15 mg. of caffeine, compared with 80 to 120 mg. in a cup of coffee. However, guarana contains other compounds that slow down the assimilation of caffeine by the body, producing a more sustained energizing effect that can last for up to six hours.

Because of its reputation as an energy enhancer, guarana is growing in popularity among athletes looking to improve their stamina and endurance. Guarana is reputed to help rid overworked muscles of lactic acid, which can pool in muscle tissue and cause post-workout aches and pains. According to anecdotal reports, guarana also helps athletes recover their strength more quickly.

For at least 400 years, guarana has been used as an herbal remedy for migraine headaches by Amazon Indians.

POSSIBLE BENEFITS

Restores energy.
May improve athletic performance.

THE RIGHT AMOUNT

Take up to three 500-mg. capsules daily. I do not recommend using guarana on a regular basis. Save it for when you really need a lift!

CAUTION

If you are pregnant, have high blood pressure, or have a heart condition, or if you want to avoid caffeine and stimulants, do not use guarana.

Gugulipid

FACTS

Extracted from the mukul myrrh tree, gugulipid has been included in the Ayurveda, the Indian system of medicine, for centuries and is officially recognized in India as a cholesterol-lowering drug. Although this herb is relatively new to the West, you can find gugulipid capsules in most natural food stores. It is also included in many combination herbal formulas for cardiovascular health.

Numerous studies, nearly all performed in India, show that gugulipid is very effective in lowering high blood cholesterol levels and high blood triglyceride levels, both of which can substantially increase the risk of heart disease and stroke. In addition, it raises the levels of HDL, or good cholesterol, offering added protection against heart disease. Gugulipid has worked as well as, or better than, many prescription cholesterol-lowering agents but without their unpleasant side effects, such as upset stomach, nausea, and possible liver damage. According to studies, gugulipid can lower cholesterol up to 27 percent, and triglycerides up to 30 percent, in a four-week period.

Gugulsterones, steroid-like compounds, are the active ingredients in gugulipid.

POSSIBLE BENEFITS

Can lower bad blood lipid levels.
Can raise HDL, or good cholesterol.

THE RIGHT AMOUNT

Take one 25-mg. gugulipid capsule with meals three times daily.

Gymnema Sylvestre

FACTS

Native to India, this herb has been used by Indian healers for nearly 2,000 years as part of the Ayurvedic traditional system of medicine. In ancient times, gymnema was known as gurmar, which literally means "sugar killer," because Ayurvedic physicians observed that chewing a few leaves from this herb suppressed the sweet taste of sugar.

For centuries, gymnema extracts have been used as a treatment for diabetes, a disorder characterized by excess sugar in the blood and urine, which can lead to serious complications ranging from stroke to blindness. Type I diabetes, which is more common among children and young adults, is caused by the inability of beta cells in the pancreas to produce enough insulin, the hormone that breaks down sugar so it can be utilized by body cells. Type II diabetes—a virtual epidemic among older Americans—may be caused by a decline in the production of insulin and/or by insulin resistance, in which the body no longer uses insulin efficiently, thereby allowing sugar levels to rise. Gymnema may be a useful treatment for both types of diabetes. Studies published in Indian journals show that it not only lowers blood sugar but may help repair damaged cells in the pancreas, the gland in which insulin is produced, thereby improving insulin production.

Although it has not been scientifically proved, gymnema is reputed to reduce the urge to eat sweets. Many people find that drinking a cup of tea with gymnema extract will make sweet things taste bitter for up to two hours. Considering that obesity is a major risk factor for diabetes and many other health problems, anything that will help shed excess pounds is a useful tool!

If you are taking medication for diabetes, consult with your physician or natural healer before using gymnema. I would also recommend this herb to people who are at high risk of developing diabetes, such as those who are overweight and are over the age of 65. If you are not diabetic but are looking to curb your sweet tooth, try taking this herb to see if it can help you beat the sugar habit.

POSSIBLE BENEFITS

Normalizes high blood sugar levels.
May put the brakes on the urge to eat sweets.

THE RIGHT AMOUNT

Gymnema sylvestre is available in capsules; take two 200-mg. capsules daily.
Gymnema extract (5–10 drops) can be mixed with tea, water, or juice; drink one cup of tea daily.

5-HTP

FACTS

5-HTP (5-hydroxytryptophan) is a new supplement that is described as the natural alternative to Prozac. Like Prozac and other drugs known as selective serotonin reuptake inhibitors (SSRIs), 5-HTP enhances the activity of serotonin, a hormone produced by the brain that is involved in mood, sleep, and appetite. Low levels of serotonin are associated with depression, anxiety, and sleep disorders. Drugs such as Prozac prevent the brain cells from using up serotonin too quickly, thereby causing a deficiency. 5-HTP works a bit differently: it increases the cell's production of serotonin, which boosts serotonin levels.

5-HTP is similar to tryptophan, another supplement that was very popular in the 1980s as a sleep aid but was recalled by the U.S. FDA in 1988 after a tainted batch from Japan caused serious side effects, including several deaths. The problem was not with the tryptophan itself but with seriously flawed manufacturing procedures. There is no evidence that 5-HTP is dangerous. In fact, the studies that I've read have led me to conclude that it may prove to be a wonderful alternative to prescription antidepressants.

For example, in one Swiss study, depressed patients were given either 100 mg. of 5-HTP three times a day or 150 mg. of fluvoxamine (an SSRI). Starting at week two and continuing through week six, both groups reported significant improvement on standard depression rating scales. However, the people taking 5-HTP seemed to have made more progress than those taking the prescription antidepressants. Other studies have shown that

5-HTP not only is an effective antidepressant but can help suppress appetite, a boon for people who need to lose weight. In fact, in one Italian study, patients taking 5-HTP reduced their carbohydrate intake and felt satisfied sooner than did a group taking a placebo.

In addition, 5-HTP has been used successfully to treat sleep disorders. Serotonin is the precursor to melatonin, the natural hormone that regulates sleep-wake cycles. When you boost your level of serotonin, you are also increasing your level of melatonin, which can result in a better night's sleep. If 5-HTP is similar to an SSRI, why not take the SSRI? For one thing, prescription antidepressants are much more expensive; for another, they often cause some unpleasant side effects, including dry mouth, anxiety, and loss of libido. These effects are not felt with 5-HTP.

POSSIBLE BENEFITS

Treats depression.
Suppresses appetite.
Helps you get a good night's sleep.

THE RIGHT AMOUNT

Take up to two 50-mg. capsules daily on an empty stomach.

Hemp Oil

FACTS

Hemp oil is a rich source of essential fatty acids, the kind of fat that is missing from the modern diet. For centuries, hemp was a major source of oil and fiber. Unfortunately, hemp oil has been unfairly maligned because the hemp plant is a member of the *Cannabis sativa* family, better known for the mind-altering drug marijuana. In fact, even though the products derived from hemp are not hallucinogenic, it is illegal to grow hemp in the U.S. Because of its important health benefits, hemp is now being imported to the U.S. from other countries, and hemp products are being sold at natural food stores.

What is so special about hemp oil? It is a wonderful source of omega-3 fatty acids, "good" fats that are required for a healthy body and mind. There are two types of essential fatty acids: omega-6 fatty acids and omega-3 fatty acids. Omega-6 fatty acids are found in nuts, seeds, avocados, grains, and most cooking oils. Most people get adequate amounts of omega-6 fatty acids through their diet, but not enough omega-3. Omega-3 oils are generally found in coldwater fatty fish, deep green vegetables, and some grains and seeds. Our hunter/gatherer ancestors had a ratio of omega-6 to omega-3 fatty acids of about 5:1. Because of modern food processing and changes in our diet, the ratio now is about 24:1. It is also very difficult to get enough omega-3 fatty acids from food alone, and to compound the problem, omega-3 fatty acids are very fragile and can be destroyed by heating.

Essential fatty acids are important because they are instrumental in many body functions: the production of hormones and the regulation of blood pressure, cholesterol, and body temperature. These fatty acids are also natural blood thinners: they can prevent blood clots, which can lead to heart attack and stroke. Essential fatty acids contain natural anti-inflammatory compounds that can relieve the symptoms of arthritis and autoimmune diseases. In addition, a diet low in essential fatty acids could result in skin problems, such as dandruff, eczema, splitting nails, and dull brittle hair. More importantly, numerous studies have shown that compounds found in essential fatty acids can block tumor formation in animals, and test tube studies have documented that omega-3 fatty acids can inhibit the growth of human breast cancer cells.

What's even more intriguing is a recent study that linked a diet low in omega-3 fatty acids to a higher incidence of depression. This is not surprising, considering that the human brain consists of more than 50 percent fat cells! Given that essential fatty acids play such a vital role in health, many researchers believe that the deficiency in omega-3 fatty acids is a leading cause of the high rates of cancer and heart disease that occurred in the second half of the twentieth century.

POSSIBLE BENEFITS

Relieves pain and inflammation of arthritis and some autoimmune problems.
May protect against heart disease.
Can block the growth of cancerous tumors.
Helps keep skin, hair, and nails healthy.
May prevent depression.

THE RIGHT AMOUNT

Hemp oil can be used in salad dressings and other foods. It has a pleasant, nutty flavor. Do not cook with hemp oil, as heat will destroy the fragile omega-3 fatty acids. Add to food after it has been cooked, or use in salad dressing.
Hemp oil capsules are easier to use. Take up to two 1000-mg. capsules daily.

HMB (Beta-hydroxy Beta-methylbutyrate)

FACTS

This new sports supplement was first developed for cattle feed by researchers at Iowa State University, but it is fast growing in popularity among two-legged animals—notably competitive athletes. HMB is a metabolite, or by-product, of the normal breakdown in the body of the amino acid leucine, which is found in plant and animal food. HMB can enhance the effects of vigorous exercise by building muscle and reducing body fat.

Clinical trials of HMB have been very promising. In one study conducted at Iowa State University, 40 men received either HMB supplements (3 grams per day) or a placebo. All of the men underwent four weeks of weight training performed three days a week. At the end of the four weeks, the group taking the HMB showed a greater increase in muscle, lost more fat, and were stronger than those not taking HMB. Because of studies like these, HMB is now being promoted as a safe alternative to anabolic steroids, which build muscle but often at a terrible cost: they are illegal and can cause serious side effects.

HMB is not a miracle pill. If you take it without working out and expect to see a difference in your body, you will be sorely disappointed. But if you use it as it is intended to be used—along with vigorous exercise—there is good evidence that you will see (and feel) some impressive results.

POSSIBLE BENEFITS

Builds muscle.
Decreases fat.

THE RIGHT AMOUNT

Take 3 grams daily in either capsule or powder form with food.

CAUTION

Pregnant or lactating women should not use HMB or any other supplement without consulting with their physicians.

Personal Advice

People have asked me whether it is safe to take creatine monohydrate with HMB. The practice of taking more than one body-building supplement is called "stacking." So far, there is no evidence that taking HMB with creatine monohydrate is harmful, and since both substances naturally occur in the body, I would assume that they can coexist peacefully.

HMP-33

FACTS

HMP-33 is a standardized ginger extract that has been used successfully in Europe to treat osteo- and rheumatoid arthritis, and is a new arrival in the United States. For centuries, ginger has been prescribed by Ayurvedic and Indian healers to treat the pain and stiffness associated with arthritis. Ginger contains natural anti-inflammatory agents called gingeroles. Fresh ginger, however, also contains compounds called shogaoles, which can cause stomach irritation in some people. HMP-33 contains a rich concentration of gingeroles but without the potentially irritating shogaoles.

HMP-33 blocks the inflammatory process in several ways. First, it inhibits the formation of prostaglandins, which are responsible for much of the pain associated with arthritis. Second, it blocks the action of leukotrines, which are involved in chronic inflammation. HMP-33 can be taken alone, or along with NSAIDs for people who need additional pain control. There are no known side effects to HMP-33. It even seems to have a protective effect on the mucous membranes in the stomach, whereas NSAIDs can cause gastric irritation. Studies performed in Copenhagen show that most patients who use HMP-33 experience significant relief in symptoms. It takes about three weeks, however, to see a real improvement. Granted, NSAIDs may work faster, but they have potentially serious side effects and cannot be used by everyone. In addition, many patients find that NSAIDs become ineffective after long-term use.

POSSIBLE BENEFITS

Relieves inflammation and pain due to osteo- and rheumatoid arthritis.
May help reduce pain due to muscle strains and injuries.
Useful for fibromyalgia and bursitis.

THE RIGHT AMOUNT

Take two capsules daily. One capsule equals 6600 mg. of dried ginger.

Hydrocitric Acid (HCA)

FACTS

If you're looking for a way to lose weight, this supplement may be just what the doctor ordered. Hydrocitric acid

(HCA) is the active ingredient extracted from the Indian fruit garcinia cambogia, a rare tropical fruit native to the jungles of Asia. A member of the tamarind family, garcinia is the size of an orange and can be either yellow or red. The sour fruit has been used in curries for hundreds of years. Recently introduced to the West, garcinia has been used for centuries by Ayurvedic healers as a digestive aid and a natural appetite suppressant.

What has captured the attention of the West is that garcinia, or more specifically HCA, may be a useful tool in the ongoing battle of the bulge. Recently, researchers have discovered that HCA is a "lipogenesis inhibitor," which means that it slows down the production of fat from the metabolism of carbohydrates and proteins. When we consume more calories than we burn, we store the excess in the form of glycogen in the liver and muscles to be used as energy as the body needs it. There is a limited amount of space for glycogen. Once our glycogen stores are filled, the excess calories are converted to fat, and the brain sends out signals telling us that we are hungry. HCA enhances the ability of the liver and muscles to store glycogen, thereby reducing fat production. At the same time, it prevents our brains from telling our stomachs that it is time to eat. The net effect is that more calories are burned as energy, fewer are turned into unwanted pounds, and we don't walk around as hungry. Animal studies have shown that HCA can suppress fat production by 40 to 80 percent for 8 to 12 hours after eating. Human studies have also confirmed that people eat less and store less body fat after taking HCA.

HCA not only is a useful weight-loss tool but may prevent heart disease by lowering high blood triglyceride levels, which are a risk factor for heart attack and stroke.

Unlike amphetamine-based over-the-counter diet pills, HCA is not habit-forming and does not cause the jitters or other unpleasant or dangerous side effects.

HCA is marketed under the trade names of Citrin and Citrimax and as HCA. It is also included in several weight-loss formulas, diet drinks, and diet bars.

Some studies suggest that HCA can reduce caloric intake by as much as 10 percent. In my experience, some people do very well on HCA—they don't eat as much, and they lose a significant amount of weight—while others don't experience any positive effects. There may be some variations in physiology that can explain the different results. If you need to lose weight, and HCA doesn't work for you, there are several other supplements you can try. Work with your physician or natural healer to find the right supplement or combination of supplements for you. However, I believe that any weight-loss supplement will be effective if you incorporate it into a sensible diet and exercise regimen.

POSSIBLE BENEFITS

May be a useful tool to help lose weight by reducing appetite. May prevent excess calories from being stored as fat.

THE RIGHT AMOUNT

Take three 500–750-mg. capsules daily. For best results, take half an hour before meals.
Drink at least eight glasses of water per day when taking this supplement.

Personal Advice

This supplement should not be used by pregnant or lactating women.

Hydroxyapatite

FACTS

Hydroxyapatite is a new form of an old favorite supplement: calcium. According to an August 1997 report issued by the National Academy of Sciences, most children and adults in the United States and Canada are getting only about half the calcium they need from food alone. Along with other minerals, calcium is required for the development and maintenance of strong bones. If you don't get enough calcium, you run the risk of developing osteoporosis, a common disease characterized by the thinning of bone, which leaves it vulnerable to fracture. More than 25 million Americans—more than two-thirds of them women—have osteoporosis.

Low-fat dairy products, such as yogurt, and to a lesser extent green leafy vegetables, such as broccoli, are good food sources of calcium. However, even though dairy foods are rich in calcium, for many people they cause problems. Although yogurt is a wonderful food, one cup provides only 300 mg. of calcium, and few people will eat more than one yogurt daily. Milk is a major cause of allergy in children, and many adults are lactose intolerant; that is, they lack an enzyme that is essential for the digestion of milk. Cheese is packed with fat, and low-fat cheese is often not a good source of calcium. As for broccoli and green vegetables, you would have to eat up to 20 servings daily (10 cups) to meet the calcium requirements. Obviously, it is impractical to rely on food sources alone to meet the daily calcium requirements.

Calcium supplements are the obvious solution, but not all calcium supplements are well absorbed by the body. Of all the calcium supplements, hydroxyapatite, made from ground-up bovine bone, is the best absorbed. Hydroxyapatite contains calcium that is identical to the calcium found in our bone, along with other minerals that are essential for strong bones, including magnesium, fluoride, sodium, and potassium. In one study published in the *American Journal of Clinical Nutrition*, 53 postmenopausal women suffering from accelerated bone loss were divided into three groups and put on different treatment regimens. All groups received monthly injections of 100,000 units of vitamin D. One group took only the vitamin D, a second group also took 1000 mg. daily of calcium gluconate, and a third group took 1000 mg. daily of hydroxyapatite. At the end of 14 months, only the group that took the hydroxyapatite showed improvement; in fact, they experienced a significant increase in bone thickness.

Supplements are not the only way to preserve bone. Weight-bearing exercise can help build bone and reduce bone loss. In addition, avoid excess caffeine intake, which can rid the body of calcium, and carbonated beverages that contain phosphorus, which in high amounts can wash calcium from the body.

POSSIBLE BENEFITS

Helps maintain strong bones and prevent osteoporosis.

THE RIGHT AMOUNT

Several supplements containing hydroxyapatite are on the market. Be sure to use one that provides 1000 mg. daily of calcium. Make up the deficit in calcium with food. If you take a hydroxyapatite supplement and eat at least one carton of nonfat yogurt daily, you will receive enough calcium.

Adolescents who are still growing require 1300 mg. of calcium daily. Up to age 50, the recommended daily intake of calcium is 1000 mg; people aged 50 and over should take 1200 mg. daily.

Personal Advice

If you are a vegetarian or prefer not to use animal products, calcium citrate is also a highly absorbable form of this mineral. I consider it a close second to hydroxyapatite.

Inositol Hexanicotinate

FACTS

Inositol hexanicotinate (IHN) is a form of niacin, the B vitamin that is well known for its ability to lower elevated blood cholesterol levels. Also called "no-flush" niacin, IHN offers all the benefits of niacin without the unpleasant or dangerous side effects associated with taking high doses of niacin, including itching, flushing, and even liver damage with long-term use. Niacin can also lower blood triglyceride levels and is one of the few supplements that can raise HDL or good cholesterol.

For obvious reasons, niacin has been promoted as a heart-healthy vitamin, but recent studies suggest that it may also be a brain-boosting vitamin. In one study, 96 people ranging in age from 35 to 85 were given several tests to assess their memory function. After taking a daily dose of 420 mg. of niacin, the subjects performed 10 to 20 percent better than when they were given a placebo. In another study performed in China, niacin was shown to protect laboratory rats from memory loss due to cerebral ischemia, the disruption of oxygen flow to the brain that is similar to what occurs in a stroke. Rats treated with niacin recovered faster and remembered previously learned tasks better than untreated rats, signifying an improvement in memory. More studies need to be done to determine if niacin can reverse memory loss due to stroke in humans, but this study is certainly promising.

POSSIBLE BENEFITS

Helps prevent heart disease by correcting abnormal blood lipids.

May enhance memory.

THE RIGHT AMOUNT

Take up to three 500-mg. capsules daily.

Kudzu

FACTS

Kudzu is the herb you wished you had taken the night before the morning after. This ancient Chinese herb, which grows wild throughout the southeastern United States, is now being promoted as the antidote to the common hangover. Kudzu contains two phytochemicals, daidzin and daidzein, which help reduce blood alcohol levels. Although clinical studies of it are scarce, an abundance of anecdotal reports suggests that kudzu supplements taken immediately before or after drinking can virtually eliminate the nausea, headache, and generally sick feeling that typically occur after a night of imbibing.

The fact that kudzu should be the treatment of choice for hangovers is not surprising. For the past 2,000 years, Asian herbalists have used a tea brewed from the kudzu root to treat alcoholism. Recently, researchers at Harvard Medical School have shown that kudzu extract can substantially reduce alcohol intake in a breed of hamsters that develop an alcohol addiction similar to that found in humans. In the study, hamsters were injected with either daidzein or daidzin and then given a choice between plain water and alcohol mixed with water. Those given either of the kudzu compounds reduced their alcohol intake by 50 percent. For reasons that are not quite understood, kudzu can reduce the desire for alcohol, and it is now being tested in this country as a treatment for alcoholism.

POSSIBLE BENEFITS

May help to break alcohol addiction.
May help prevent or relieve hangovers.

THE RIGHT AMOUNT

Take up to three 500-mg. capsules daily before or after drinking alcohol.

Lactoferrin

FACTS

At the turn of the century, the average life span was a mere 47 years, and infection was the most common cause of death. Thanks to improved nutrition, better hygiene, and, of course, antibiotics, we have managed to add more than three decades to the average life span. Certainly, we owe a debt to penicillin and other wonder drugs that helped us survive potentially deadly infections such as pneumonia and strep.

As we approach a new millennium, however, we are faced with a new challenge. Although antibiotics have saved countless lives, they have outlived their usefulness in many ways. As I have noted earlier, the overuse of antibiotics has created new "monster" strains of bacteria that are resistant to even the strongest drugs. As a result, drug-resistant staph infections are rampant throughout hospitals in the United States. And for many common conditions, such as ear infections in children, antibiotics have been rendered useless. Obviously, we need to find new ways to fight bacterial infections that will not create even bigger problems down the road. If we are more sparing in our use of antibiotics, they will be effective when we really do need them.

Lactoferrin, a supplement new to natural food stores, is a giant leap in the right direction. A protein that is abundant in breast milk, lactoferrin plays a role in helping infants maintain a healthy balance of "friendly" bacteria in their intestines. This is important because friendly bacteria control the growth and activity of disease-carrying bacteria. Lactoferrin attacks harmful bacteria in several ways. First, it penetrates the protective cell membrane of bacteria, making it impossible for the bacteria to reproduce. Second, it "starves" the bacteria by binding with excess iron, depriving the bacteria of a nutrient it needs for growth. Finally, unlike antibiotics that indiscriminately kill both good and bad bacteria, lactoferrin actually enhances the levels of good bacteria in the body.

Lactoferrin is used in Japan by pediatricians to treat ear infections. Cutting-edge alternative physicians in the United States are already prescribing lactoferrin to patients with weakened immune systems, such as cancer patients undergoing chemotherapy. According to one small study in Europe, chemotherapy patients given lactoferrin had fewer negative side effects, such as diarrhea, than patients not given lactoferrin.

For the best results, take lactoferrin at the first sign of illness. For broader protection, take lactoferrin with an antiviral supplement, such as monolaurin (see page 111).

Although lactoferrin supplements are derived from cow's milk, lactoferrin is sterilized and refined and should not cause any allergic reactions. Researchers are working on developing a recombinant form of human lactoferrin made from cloning, which is believed to work even better than bovine lactoferrin.

POSSIBLE BENEFITS

Acts as a natural antibiotic.
Kills infections without harming friendly bacteria.

THE RIGHT AMOUNT

Lactoferrin is available in capsules and chewable wafers. Take two 250-mg. capsules or wafers daily for up to two weeks.

L-Carnitine

FACTS

This supplement promises to make you stronger, sleeker, and healthier. L-carnitine is a vitamin-like nutrient that is found in the heart, brain, and skeletal muscles. Its primary job is to transport fatty acids across the cell wall to the mitochondria, the powerhouse of the cell, providing heart and skeletal cells with energy. For the past two decades, I have been reporting on L-carnitine as a potential treatment for coronary artery disease (CAD), in which one or more arteries delivering blood to the heart has narrowed, thereby reducing the amount of oxygen getting to the heart. L-carnitine is especially helpful for CAD because it enables the heart to use its limited oxygen supply more efficiently. In fact, several studies have shown that heart patients who take L-carnitine supplements can exercise longer and harder without experiencing chest pain. To add to its heart-healthy benefits, L-carnitine can also lower high blood cholesterol levels while boosting levels of beneficial HDL, the good cholesterol.

Recently, L-carnitine has been promoted as a sports supplement that can increase physical stamina and promote weight loss. Studies of the effectiveness of L-carnitine as a sports supplement have been mixed; some show that L-carnitine can dramatically improve aerobic ability and athletic performance, whereas others have been disappointing. There is a great deal of anecdotal evidence, however, attesting to the ability of L-carnitine to increase energy, and many people swear that it has made a real difference in how they feel and in their ability to work out. If you are interested, you can try it and see if it works as well for you.

Italian researchers report that L-carnitine can help increase the effectiveness of sperm in men with infertility problems. In one study, 47 men with a normal sperm count, but whose sperm showed poor motility (low activity), were given 1 gram of L-carnitine three times daily for three months. At the end of the study, 37 men showed improvement in sperm motility, which would increase the likelihood that the sperm would be able to fertilize an egg.

L-carnitine is also being promoted as a supplement that can prevent or reverse some of the symptoms associated with Alzheimer's disease or aging. In test tube studies and animal studies, L-carnitine was able to reverse much of the damage inflicted to brain cells by free radicals, which is typical of the kind of damage seen in the brains of Alzheimer's patients. According to several Italian studies, L-carnitine supplements can slow down the rate of mental deterioration in patients diagnosed with Alzheimer's disease on the basis of standard mental assessment tests. Other Italian studies performed on the mildly impaired elderly showed that L-carnitine helped improve memory in older people. These positive results have not been duplicated in similar studies performed in the United States, so the jury is still out on the effectiveness of L-carnitine for this purpose.

POSSIBLE BENEFITS

Helps improve oxygen utilization in heart patients.
Enhances athletic performance and strength.
May protect against Alzheimer's disease, or slow its progress.

THE RIGHT AMOUNT

Take up to three 250- to 500-mg. capsules or tablets daily, half an hour before eating or two hours after eating.

Lipoic Acid

FACTS

Dubbed the "universal antioxidant," lipoic acid, which has only just begun to appear on the shelves of health food stores, is a vitamin-like substance that is naturally produced in the body. Lipoic acid plays a unique role in defending the body against free radical attack, and it is widely used as a treatment for diabetes in Europe. As we age we stop producing lipoic acid in sufficient quantities, which is why we need to take supplements.

Dr. Lester Packer, a world-renowned scientist who heads the Membrane Bioenergetics Group at the University of California at Berkeley, is the world's leading authority on lipoic acid and antioxidants. Dr. Packer discovered that unlike other antioxidants that have a specific job in the body, lipoic acid can serve as a "free agent" that can pinch-hit for the other antioxidants when they are in short supply. In other words, if you are low in vitamins E or C, lipoic acid will temporarily take over their jobs. Lipoic acid also greatly enhances the potency of vitamins C and E.

In one fascinating study from Dr. Packer's laboratory, three groups of 12-week-old mice were given different diets. One group was given a normal diet; the second was given a vitamin E-deficient diet, and the third was given a vitamin E-deficient diet but supplemented with lipoic acid. The animals in the first group developed normally, but the animals in the second group (the vitamin E-deficient group without lipoic acid) developed severe wasting syndrome and seemed to shrivel up. But the animals in the vitamin E-deficient group that were given lipoic acid supplements developed normally and showed none of the signs of vitamin E deficiency. Clearly, lipoic acid spared them from the ravages of vitamin E deficiency.

More than two decades ago, Burton Berkson, M.D., at the National Institutes of Health, discovered that lipoic acid could cure a fatal liver disease caused by the ingestion of amanita mushrooms, which are highly poisonous. Amanita mushrooms inflict their damage by promoting the formation of toxic free radicals that rapidly destroy liver cells. Sixty to 90 percent of people who eat this dangerous mushroom die; yet, scientists found that lipoic acid cured these patients.

One of the most important functions of lipoic acid is to normalize blood sugar levels. High blood sugar is a common problem for many middle-aged and older men and women because they develop insulin resistance (also known as Type II diabetes), a condition that affects some 16 million Americans. Insulin is the hormone that helps break down sugar or glucose so it can be utilized by the body's cells. If you are resistant to insulin, you will have higher than normal levels of blood sugar, or glucose, and over time, these high levels can result in serious health problems such as atherosclerosis (hardening of the arteries), nerve damage, and blindness. Lipoic acid has been used quite successfully in Europe for several decades to prevent complications from insulin resistance and other forms of diabetes, but it has been virtually ignored in the United States.

Recently, body builders have discovered the power of lipoic acid. When you exercise, your body requires more oxygen to produce energy. The more oxygen you use, the more likely you are to produce free radicals, which can cause the sore, stiff feeling that often accompanies a rigorous workout. People who work out tell me that since they've been taking lipoic acid, they do not feel as sore and uncomfortable the day after.

There is even more exciting news from Dr. Packer's lab. Recently, lipoic acid was able to completely reverse damage caused by stroke (the deprivation of blood to the brain) in animals. In human beings, stroke not only is a leading of cause of death but can inflict severe brain damage, leaving its victims paralyzed. There is no known cure for stroke, but if lipoic acid works as well in humans as it does in animals, it could provide an effective treatment that may minimize damage.

POSSIBLE BENEFITS

Protects against free radical damage.
Can prevent serious complications from diabetes.
May enhance ability to work out.
Has potential as a treatment for stroke.

THE RIGHT AMOUNT

Lipoic acid is available in tablets and is included in antioxidant formulas. Take up to two 50-mg. tablets daily.

Lutein

FACTS

Do you eat three cups of chopped spinach or collard greens every day? If you do, then you don't need this supplement. If, however, you're like most folks, you'd better keep on reading.

Lutein is a cutting-edge new supplement that could make the difference between maintaining your vision well into old age, or going blind. The most common cause of blindness in people 65 and over is age-related macular degeneration, a condition caused by the destruction of the macula, the small central part of the retina. The macula is responsible for central vision, the kind that is necessary for activities such as recognizing faces, reading, writing, and driving your car. As many as 20 percent of all people 65 and older suffer from macular degeneration. There is a 500 percent increased risk among postmenopausal women, which is believed to be due in part to the decline in estrogen. Although the precise cause of macular degeneration is unknown, constant exposure to ultraviolet light from the sun, which can promote the formation of free radicals, is a likely suspect.

There is no cure for macular degeneration, but in some cases, laser surgery may help slow down the progress of the disease. There is also compelling evidence that eating the right food and taking the right supplements can offer significant protection. Lutein is a member of the carotenoid family and is found in vegetables such as spinach, kale, collard greens, mustard greens, and corn. There is a high concentration of lutein in the macula, which prompted researchers to investigate whether the lutein in food had any effect on vision. In one well-known study performed at Harvard, researchers investigated the dietary intake of a variety of carotenoids, including lutein, in relation to the risk of developing macular degeneration. The study revealed that people who consumed at least 6 grams of lutein daily from their diet had a much lower incidence of macular degeneration than those who did not.

The problem, as I mentioned earlier, is that not everyone eats enough lutein-rich food, and until recently, lutein supplements were not available. In fact, lutein had long been ignored, because unlike more famous carotenoids such as beta carotene, it did not convert to vitamin A in the body and was therefore considered useless. We now know that lutein is an antioxidant; some researchers speculate that it may deactivate dangerous free radicals caused by harmful ultraviolet rays, and thereby protect the eyes from oxidative damage. Fortunately, there are now dozens of lutein products to choose from, including numerous combination formulas especially designed to improve vision. Most of these combination products include zinc, a mineral that is also involved in the maintenance of the macula, and zeaxanthin (see page 176), another carotenoid found in the macula.

POSSIBLE BENEFITS

Prevents macular degeneration; preserves vision.

THE RIGHT AMOUNT

Lutein is available in tablets and combination products. Take one 6- to 20-mg. tablet daily. (If you buy a combination that includes other supplements, be sure that it contains at least 6 mg. of lutein.)

Lycopene

FACTS

Lycopene is one of the 600 or so members of the carotenoid family, phytochemicals that are abundant in fruits and vegetables. The best food sources of lycopene are tomato and tomato products. In fact, lycopene is the primary carotenoid consumed by Americans.

Beta carotene, the most famous of the carotenoids, has long intrigued researchers because of its pro-vitamin A activity—that is, it is converted to vitamin A as the body needs it. Much research has been done on beta carotene, but lesser-known carotenoids such as lycopene, which do not have any pro-vitamin A activity, have long been ignored. Until very recently it was believed that these "junk" carotenoids served little purpose other than to color food. More careful investigation, however, has shed new light on the unique role of carotenoids such as lycopene. In fact, researchers now believe that lycopene is a more potent antioxidant than beta carotene and also a powerful anticancer agent. For example, you may recall an intriguing study that showed that men who ate the most pizza had much lower rates of prostate cancer than those who did not. What you may not know, however, is that the reduced risk of prostate cancer is believed to be due to the lycopene-rich tomato sauce.

Since that groundbreaking study, researchers have tested lycopene on human and animal cancer cells, and the results have been very promising. Researchers at the Ben-Gurion University and Soroka Medical Center in Israel have reported that lycopene inhibited the growth of cancer cells from breast, lung, and endometrial cancers. What's even more remarkable is that when laboratory animals were fed potent carcinogens, high levels of lycopene helped to suppress cancerous growths. In fact, the higher the dose of lycopene, the more effective it was against cancer. Lycopene is particularly effective against the chemical carcinogens found in tobacco smoke. Another recent study suggests that lycopene may help protect skin against damage from exposure to ultraviolet light, which can cause wrinkles and even skin cancer.

Since blood levels of lycopene decline with age, this is one supplement you should consider if you are 50 or older, especially if you do not consume at least one tomato product daily. By the way, simply drinking a glass of tomato juice or eating a fresh tomato is not enough. The lycopene in tomato is not well absorbed by the body unless it is heated and combined with a small amount of fat, such as olive oil.

POSSIBLE BENEFITS

Appears to reduce the risk of prostate cancer.
May protect against many different types of cancers, including breast and skin cancer.

THE RIGHT AMOUNT

Take one 6- to 10-mg. capsule daily with meals.

Lysine

FACTS

Lysine is one of the eight essential amino acids that cannot be produced by the body but must be obtained from food, such as meat, fish, milk, and cheese. For more than a decade, lysine has been prescribed by natural healers and mainstream physicians to treat cold sores and other symptoms caused by the herpes simplex-1 virus, which can lie dormant for years and recur without warning. Recently, however, researchers have uncovered some new and fascinating uses for lysine.

Dr. Linus Pauling, best known for his work with vitamin C, also investigated the use of lysine as a treatment for angina, chest pain due to oxygen deprivation. In one small study, Pauling gave three patients up to 6 grams of lysine supplements daily in divided doses. Two of the patients had already undergone coronary bypass surgery, all of them were experiencing chest pain on exertion, and all relied on sublingual nitroglycerin tablets to control pain. Within two to four weeks after taking lysine, all three patients had improved so much that they were able to eliminate their sublingual nitroglycerin tablets. Even better, they were able to increase their exercise, which would help their hearts mend all the faster. Other studies have shown that lysine can lower high blood pressure and elevated triglyceride levels, which would be beneficial both to heart patients and to people at risk of developing heart disease. If you have angina, you may want to talk to your physician or natural healer about using lysine to control your symptoms.

Lysine also may be an important supplement for menopausal women. Once women reach menopause, they are at greater risk of developing osteoporosis, a disease characterized by the thinning of bone, leaving them vulnerable to breaks and fractures. Lysine may help preserve bone by enabling the body to use calcium more efficiently. Although it is not a cure for osteoporosis, lysine may be one more important tool in preventing it. Also, lysine is instrumental in the formation of collagen, the underlying tissue that provides the scaffolding that supports the outer layer of skin. Since as we age, we lose collagen, our skin wrinkles and sags. Although both men and women experience this change, in women it is exacerbated by the decline in estrogen, which helps the skin retain moisture and is involved in collagen production. Lysine supplements can help keep skin looking and feeling younger.

POSSIBLE BENEFITS

Helps alleviate symptoms of herpes infection and helps prevent recurrence.
May be a useful treatment for angina.
Helps promote bone growth and healthy skin.

THE RIGHT AMOUNT

Lysine is available in capsules and tablets. To prevent a recurrence of herpes, take 500 to 1000 mg. daily.
For angina, check with your physician or natural healer.
For better skin and stronger bones, take 500 mg. daily.

Maitake Mushroom Extract

FACTS

Maitake mushroom, grown in northern Japan, has been revered for centuries for its delicate flavor and unique medicinal properties. Today, maitake mushroom extract is highly prized for its cancer-fighting and immune-boosting benefits. *Maitake* literally means "dancing mushroom" because legend has it that when mushroom hunters found this rare, gourmet delight in the mountains of Japan, they would dance for joy. Maitake mushrooms can grow up to 20 inches in diameter and can weigh up to 100 pounds. During feudal times, maitake mushrooms were literally worth their weight in silver and were used as currency.

In the 1980s, Japanese researchers began to investigate the folklore behind medicinal mushrooms and found that many had truly remarkable properties. For example, maitake mushroom stimulates the immune system by activating T-cells, the body's natural defenders against viruses and cancer cells. Recent animal studies have shown that maitake extract can shrink tumors in mice even better than a common chemotherapy drug. What is truly remarkable is that when maitake extract was combined with the chemotherapy drug, there was a 99 percent tumor shrinkage within 14 days—a considerably shorter period than when the drug was used alone. Double-blind studies on maitake extract are under way at the Cancer Treatment Centers of America involving patients with advanced colorectal cancer receiving chemotherapy. Maitake not only enhances the effectiveness of chemotherapy but also appears to reduce some of its unwanted side effects, such as nausea and extreme fatigue.

As you probably know, the HIV virus, which causes AIDS, specifically targets disease-fighting T-cells, leaving the body defenseless against infection. Studies conducted by both the Japan National Institute of Health and the U.S. National Cancer Institute have verified that maitake extract can prevent the destruction of T-cells by HIV as much as 97 percent. In fact, some physicians are already using maitake extract successfully along with other therapies for AIDS patients.

Maitake is not only useful in illness but can fortify the immune system so that you can resist disease in the first place.

POSSIBLE BENEFITS

Strengthens immune function.
May work as an effective cancer therapy alone or in combination with chemotherapy drugs.

THE RIGHT AMOUNT

Take one 100-mg. standardized tablet daily.

Malic Acid

FACTS

Malic acid is one of many alpha hydroxy acids (AHAs) found in fruits and vegetables including apples, grapes and cranberries. In recent years, alpha-hydroxy acids have gained popularity for external use as skin exfoliants, but what you may not know is that one AHA, malic acid, plays a critical role internally for normal energy production.

Malic acid is believed to be instrumental in preventing hypoxia, a breakdown in the delivery of oxygen to muscle cells that can cause muscles to fatigue easily. In this regard, malic acid has been tested as a treatment for fibromyalgia, a condition characterized by chronic exhaustion as well as unspecified aches and pains, which may be related to hypoxia. There is no cure for fibromyalgia, and few treatments are effective. For reasons unknown, fibromyalgia primarily affects women. In one study published in the *Journal of Nutritional Medicine*, 15 fibromyalgia patients were given either 1200 to 2400 mg. of malic acid daily with 300 to 600 mg. of magnesium for 4 to 6 weeks, or a placebo. All the patients reported a marked decrease in pain within two days, which continued throughout the time they were receiving malic acid. When the women were switched over to the placebo, however, their condition deteriorated within 48 hours. This study encourages researchers to hope that malic acid may be a breakthrough in the treatment of fibromyalgia, and perhaps of other ailments that could be due to hypoxia, such as chronic fatigue syndrome.

Athletes hope that malic acid will prove to be a supplement that can improve stamina and endurance. They have reason to be hopeful. Animal studies have shown that malic acid can enhance energy production and improve aerobic capacity. Given the important role of malic acid in helping to prevent oxygen deficiency in muscles, it stands to reason that it may maximize energy production and improve athletic performance.

POSSIBLE BENEFITS

Can relieve symptoms of fibromyalgia.
May improve endurance.

THE RIGHT AMOUNT

Take up to two 200-mg. tablets daily, one hour before eating and at bedtime.

Medium-Chain Triglycerides (MCTs)

FACTS

Eat more fat to lose fat? Sounds improbable, but it's not— as long as you're eating the right kind of fat. Medium-chain triglycerides (MCTs) are saturated fats derived from coconut oil. You may have heard that saturated fat is to be avoided at all cost because it is unhealthy. What is not widely known is that there are several different kinds of saturated fats, and some may actually be beneficial. MCTs are a case in point. Unlike other types of bad saturated fat, which put weight on you and raise blood cholesterol levels, MCTs are rapidly burned by the body and therefore do not promote weight gain or raise blood cholesterol levels. Second, because they are burned so fast, they provide a wonderful energy boost. (As of this writing, one new study suggested that MCTs may raise levels of LDL cholesterol. Therefore, I do not recommend MCTs for people with cholesterol problems.)

Some studies show that MCTs have a thermogenic effect; that is, they can stimulate the body to burn calories faster. Not surprisingly, MCT oil and capsules are becoming popular among two groups: athletes and dieters. Athletes use MCTs for additional energy to fuel their workouts. In addition, MCTs are believed to have a protein-sparing effect; that is, they burn fat but spare muscle.

MCTs combined with carbohydrates may have a synergistic effect that can enhance athletic performance. In one South African study, trained cyclists who drank a combination MCT/carbohydrate sport drink before and during their ride, at 10-minute intervals, shaved more than 5 minutes off the time they took to complete a 40-kilometer ride, compared with the results when they drank a plain carbohydrate drink or a plain MCT drink. Researchers speculate that adding the MCT to the carbohydrates prevents the muscles from rapidly depleting their carbohydrate stores, which leads to fatigue.

MCT oil should not be used in cooking, but it can be added to food or used as a spread or in salad dressing.

POSSIBLE BENEFITS

Helps shed unwanted pounds.
Provides a good source of energy.

Lowers blood cholesterol.
Improves athletic endurance.

THE RIGHT AMOUNT

Take 2 tablespoons of MCT up to two to four times daily.
Take up to two 500-mg. tablets daily, before meals or
   exercising.

CAUTION

MCTs should not be used by people with diabetes or with elevated blood cholesterol levels.

Melatonin

FACTS

Melatonin is a natural hormone produced by the pineal gland, a pea-sized structure embedded deep within the brain. Melatonin production peaks at night during sleep and falls during the day. The daily ebb and flow of melatonin controls the body's sleep/wake cycles. For years, I have been recommending melatonin as an occasional sleep aid for insomnia and as a treatment for jet lag.

Recently, melatonin has been promoted as an anti-aging supplement, because as we age, our levels of melatonin steadily decline. Animal studies have shown that adding melatonin to the drinking water of older animals can not only significantly extend life but reverse many of the telltale signs of aging. On the basis of these studies, some researchers believe that restoring youthful levels of melatonin in humans could help prevent or slow down age-related declines in physical and mental function. Countless numbers of baby boomers who are looking for ways to turn back the aging clock are now taking melatonin daily. Time will tell whether or not this hormone affects the aging process, but in the meantime, there are some other fascinating new findings about melatonin.

Melatonin is a potent antioxidant and free radical scavenger that can protect cells from oxidative damage. Oxidative damage contributes to many different diseases, including Alzheimer's disease, which is characterized by the formation of amyloid plaques in the brain that can kill brain cells. According to a report recently published in the *Journal of Neuroscience*, melatonin has been shown in test tube studies to inhibit the oxidative damage that can lead to amyloid formation in the brain, which suggests that it may help to prevent Alzheimer's.

Another new study showed that melatonin helps relieve cluster headaches, particularly debilitating headaches that primarily affect men. In a small double-blind controlled study, 20 cluster headache patients were given either 10 mg. of melatonin daily or a placebo. Half of the melatonin treatment group noticed a marked improvement after about one month of treatment, as opposed to no improvement in the placebo group. If you suffer from cluster headaches, talk to your physician or natural healer about using melatonin.

For some time, it's been known that melatonin can boost immune function by activating the cancer-fighting cells that weed out potential malignancies before they can spread. An exciting report published in the *Journal of Pineal Research* suggests that melatonin may help extend the life of patients with melanoma, a serious form of skin cancer, who were treated surgically for cancer node recurrence—a sign that the disease has metastasized, or spread to other cells. The study included 30 patients who received either 20 mg. of melatonin nightly or no treatment. After 31 months, the researchers noted that the survival rate in the melatonin group was considerably better than in those not receiving treatment.

POSSIBLE BENEFITS

Treats for jet lag and insomnia.
Has potential antiaging properties.
May help prevent Alzheimer's disease.
Reduces incidence of cluster headaches.
Activates cancer-fighting immune cells.

THE RIGHT AMOUNT

For insomnia, take 1 to 5 mg. of melatonin before bedtime. Start with 1 mg., and if that doesn't work, increase the dose by 1 mg. for a maximum of 5 mg. For best results, use the sublingual form, which dissolves under the tongue.

For jet lag, take 1 to 3 mg. in sublingual tablet form about half an hour before you want to go to sleep in your new destination.

For general antiaging benefits, take 0.5 to 1 mg. in sublingual tablet form before bedtime.

CAUTIONS

Melatonin will make you very sleepy, so take it only before going to bed. Needless to say, do not drive or operate heavy machinery after taking melatonin. In rare cases, melatonin may interact with prescription medications. If you are taking any medication, especially tranquilizers, talk to your doctor before using melatonin. In addition, if you have an autoimmune disease, do not take melatonin, since it may overstimulate immune function.

Modified Citrus Pectin

FACTS

Thousands of years ago, Chinese healers applied citrus peel to breast tumors. Today, this folk treatment is being investigated by some of the world's top cancer researchers, and preliminary studies confirm that these ancient healers knew precisely what they were doing.

Citrus peel—or actually the white pulpy stuff that we typically discard before eating—contains pectin, a carbohydrate found in plant cell walls. Citrus fruits, such as oranges, lemons, and grapefruits, are an especially rich source of pectin. Modified citrus pectin (MCP), more potent and absorbable than regular pectin, can substantially slow down the spread of cancerous cells and is particularly effective against hard-to-treat cancers such as melanoma and prostate cancer. According to one report published in the *Journal of the National Cancer Institute,* researchers found that MCP could prevent the spread of melanoma in mice, a particularly deadly form of skin cancer. Other studies have shown that MCP can thwart the spread of prostate, breast, and lung cancer in animals.

The good news is that MCP works just as well in human cancer cells, at least in test tube studies. These early results have been so encouraging that studies involving human cancer patients are under way. However, several cutting-edge physicians in the United States are already using MCP to treat cancer patients. Researchers speculate that MCP may bind to cancer cells and interfere with their ability to attach to the new blood vessels that are necessary to support new cells. Without access to new blood vessels, the cancerous cells cannot spread, or metastasize.

Nutritionists estimate that you'd have to eat the equivalent of three whole grapefruits daily, pulp and all, to consume enough pectin to protect against cancer. But you don't have to, now that MCP is available in powder and capsule form.

POSSIBLE BENEFITS

Can slow down the spread of cancer.

THE RIGHT AMOUNT

Take up to 15 grams of MCP daily in capsules or powder.

Monolaurin

FACTS

Breast-fed infants are usually healthier and stronger than bottle-fed infants because they are protected by special compounds in breast milk that help fight against infection and enhance immune function. For example, lauric acid, a fatty acid found in breast milk and marketed under the name of monolaurin, has strong antiviral properties.

Resistant to antibiotics, viruses are particularly difficult to control. Unlike bacteria, which can reproduce on their own, viruses can reproduce only after they attach themselves to other cells in our bodies and take over the functions of those cells. Obviously, in order to stop the virus, you need to prevent it from reproducing, but you don't want to kill healthy cells in the process. In numerous test tube studies, monolaurin has been shown to selectively inhibit viral replication without destroying healthy cells. For more than a decade, alternative physicians have used monolaurin to treat chronic fatigue syndrome, infections related to Epstein-Barr virus and herpes I and II virus, and flu-like symptoms with some success, in combination with high doses of vitamin C.

Monolaurin is now available for consumers in natural food stores and through mail order. It is not a supplement for daily use but should be reserved for those times when you are experiencing cold and flu symptoms. For best results, take monolaurin at the first sign of muscle ache, sore throat, headache, swollen glands, and other symptoms of viral infection.

Although monolaurin is on the cutting edge of antiviral supplements, fatty acids have been used since biblical times to treat viruses. Lauric acid is nontoxic and is on the U.S. FDA list of food additives generally recognized as safe (GRAS). For herpes infection, monolaurin is usually combined with lysine (see page 100) amino acid.

POSSIBLE BENEFITS

Helps fight viral infections.

THE RIGHT AMOUNT

At the sign of infection, take three to six 100-mg. capsules daily on an empty stomach for 14 days.

Methylsulfonylmethane (MSM)

FACTS

About 2,000 years ago, Hippocrates, known as the father of modern medicine, used sulfur fumes from garlic to treat many different diseases, including cancer. Sulfur, a nonmetallic mineral, is found in virtually every cell of the body and is essential for nearly every bodily function. Only recently have we begun to rediscover the power of sulfur, particularly one form of organic sulfur: MSM, which is easily absorbed by the body. (Do not confuse organic sulfur, which is nonallergenic, with the synthetic *sulfa* drugs, which can trigger allergic reactions in many people.)

MSM is found in plants, meat, eggs, poultry, and dairy foods. It is used by the body to make important enzymes, antibodies, glutathione (the body's main antioxidant), and connective tissue, such as cartilage, collagen, hair, nails, and skin. MSM is critical for the production of amino acids, the building blocks that make protein. Without MSM and other sulfur compounds, protein cannot hold its molecular structure. It is difficult to get enough MSM through food, however, since it is often destroyed during processing. On the basis of numerous studies on the role of MSM in the body, I believe that even a mild MSM deficiency can contribute to many medical problems, either directly or indirectly.

Several studies have documented the potential of MSM as a treatment for a wide variety of ailments. MSM is particularly effective in relieving severe allergic symptoms and asthma. In fact, I have recommended MSM along with vitamin C and other bioflavonoids to several allergy sufferers, and the results have been nothing short of amazing. Within two or three weeks, the annoying symptoms, such as runny nose and watery eyes, simply disappeared, even at the height of hay fever season.

MSM is also an effective treatment for arthritis, which is caused by the wearing away of cartilage, the substance that cushions bones. I recommend using MSM with another sulfur compound, glucosamine (see page 63), which has recently been touted as the "arthritis cure"; the two "sulfur sisters" work especially well together. People report that the supplements can significantly reduce the pain, stiffness, and tenderness typical of arthritis.

MSM is also important for wound healing: It promotes the formation of collagen, which helps produce new skin. People who take MSM also report that it can strengthen their hair and nails and is especially good for brittle, peeling nails. I can tell you from personal experience that it makes hair thicker and shinier.

POSSIBLE BENEFITS

Reduces allergic symptoms.
Relieves pain and inflammation from arthritis.
Promotes wound healing.

THE RIGHT AMOUNT

MSM is sold as tablets or a skin lotion.
Take two 1000-mg. tablets daily with food.
Apply lotion to skin one to three times daily.

Personal Advice

The tablet I take has a C-bioflavonoid complex plus 1000 mg. MSM for better absorption. For allergies, parasitic infections, and faster recovery after working out, MSM can't be beat.

N-Acetyl Cysteine (NAC)

FACTS

N-acetyl cysteine (NAC) is an exciting new supplement that can benefit everyone from body builders to the chronically ill. NAC is an amino acid that is a precursor to glutathione, the body's most abundant antioxidant, which is found in virtually every cell.

NAC has been extensively studied as a potential treatment for chemically induced cancers and for respiratory problems. In fact, studies are currently under way at the National Cancer Institute in the United States and the EUROSCAN project in Europe designed to identify safe, effective, and economical cancer treatments. Preliminary results have been extremely promising. Animal studies have shown that NAC can prevent damaging changes to DNA (the genetic material within the cell) caused by chemicals in cigarette smoke that promote the formation of free radicals, thereby triggering the growth of cancerous cells. In one study, rats exposed to cigarette smoke but given NAC did not develop the expected changes in DNA in such vulnerable sites as their lungs or trachea, two areas that are highly susceptible to injury if they are constantly exposed to cigarette smoke. NAC boosts the levels of glutathione in lung tissue, which helps protect cells against damage inflicted by free radicals. If you smoke now or have ever smoked, you should consider taking this supplement. (And of course, you should quit smoking!)

Free radical damage extends far beyond cancer. It is now believed to be a major cause of many different ailments, including chronic respiratory diseases. Numerous human studies have shown that NAC can help prevent such ailments as bronchitis, bronchial asthma, emphysema, and chronic sinusitis. In one important study, more than 2,500 patients with severe respiratory ailments were given a daily dose of 600 mg. of NAC. In most patients, lung capacity improved significantly, and coughing and mucus production were reduced. NAC can also boost immune function by activating important cells that help fight unwanted invaders. Interestingly, fewer disease-causing bacteria were found in the bronchial pathways of people who took NAC, which underscores its protective effect. And numerous people who are prone to develop lung infections swear that taking NAC daily has helped to keep them well.

NAC has also been used successfully on people with serious inner ear infections. In most cases, ear infections clear up on their own; sometimes, fluid remains in the inner ear for months and hearing can be affected. In addition, the overuse of antibiotics for ear infections in children has given rise to new strains of drug-resistant bacteria that are unresponsive to antibiotic therapy and are extremely difficult to treat. NAC is an alternative treatment for ear infections that may be safer and more effective than current treatment.

Body builders take NAC to help them recover faster from their workouts. After vigorous exercise, there is an increase in blood levels of free radicals, which is why muscles feel sore and stiff, and a decrease in available glutathione, which has been used to mop up free radicals. Studies show that supplemental NAC can replenish blood levels of glutathione, which in turn will reduce the level of free radicals in the blood and promote a quicker recovery.

POSSIBLE BENEFITS

Protects against cancer-causing chemicals in cigarette smoke.
Increases levels of glutathione.
May prevent lung infections.
Helps treat ear infections.
Speeds recovery after exercise.

THE RIGHT AMOUNT

Take three 500-mg. capsules or tablets of NAC with meals.

CAUTION

Do not use if you have peptic ulcers, or use drugs known to cause gastric lesions.

Personal Advice

If you are plagued with sinus headaches, try taking NAC. It will help relieve the sinusitis that is causing the headache.

If you suffer from recurrent respiratory or ear infections, talk to your physician or natural healer about taking NAC.

Nicotininamide Adenine Dinucleotide (NADH)

FACTS

In recent years, there has been a growing interest in the role of antioxidants for health in general, and a greater focus on some of the lesser known antioxidants in particular. One of those newly discovered antioxidants is lipoic acid (see page 94); another is NADH, also known as coenzyme-1. Enzymes are proteins that bring about chemical changes; like other coenzymes, NADH works with enzymes to produce literally thousands of biochemical reactions within the body.

NADH, a derivative of niacin, is found in all living cells and plays a vital role in energy production, particularly in the brain and nervous system. The more NADH, the greater the capacity of cells to produce energy. As we age, our levels of NADH decline, as do levels of other important antioxidants. Many researchers believe that the loss of NADH may promote diseases normally associated with brain aging, such as Alzheimer's disease and Parkinson's disease. In addition, low levels of NADH may be a contributing factor in depression and chronic fatigue syndrome.

Recently, some very exciting studies on NADH have attracted the attention of the medical community worldwide. In one study conducted at the famous Birkmayer Institute for Parkinson's Therapy in Vienna, 885 patients with Parkinson's disease were given NADH either orally or intravenously. A potentially crippling disease, Parkinson's is known by the characteristic twitches and muscle spasms that can severely hamper mobility in people affected by it. There is no cure, and effective treatments are few, but NADH offers some hope. About 80 percent of the Parkinson's patients who were given NADH showed improvement, and 20 percent responded extremely well. More specifically, NADH appeared to help reduce some of the depressive symptoms normally associated with Parkinson's.

NADH has also been used to treat Alzheimer's disease, a degenerative disease of the brain that primarily afflicts older people. Levels of NADH are 20 to 50 percent lower in Alzheimer's patients than in people of the same age who remain free of Alzheimer's. In another study, Alzheimer's patients given 10 mg. NADH daily showed a noticeable improvement in cognitive function and memory. The researchers cautioned, however, that a larger, double-blind study was needed to determine whether NADH is really helpful. Such a study on Alzheimer's patients is under way at Georgetown University Medical Center in Washington, D.C. In addition, researchers at Georgetown will also be testing NADH on patients with chronic fatigue syndrome, a condition with no known cause that is defined as prolonged exhaustion that cannot be relieved by rest and does not result from other medical problems. Up to 6 percent of the United States population is believed to suffer from chronic fatigue syndrome.

Any supplement that promises to energize the body is going to be embraced by the fitness crowd, and NADH is no exception. There are anecdotal reports from athletes that NADH makes them feel stronger and more energized. In fact, there is an ongoing study at the Nicholas Sports Institute at Lenox Hill Hospital in New York to investigate whether NADH can enhance strength and stamina in competitive athletes.

Healthy people who take NADH as a daily supplement report feeling smarter and more alert. NADH could turn out to be the supplement for both brain and brawn!

POSSIBLE BENEFITS

Protects against brain aging.
Relieves symptoms of Alzheimer's and Parkinson's diseases.
Enhances ability to work out.
May increase memory and ability to concentrate.

THE RIGHT AMOUNT

Take up to two 5-mg. tablets daily on an empty stomach.

Natural Progesterone

FACTS

As 50 million baby boomers reach midlife—more than half of them women—products designed to ease the symptoms of menopause are dominating the shelves of pharmacies and natural food stores. Natural progesterone cream is one of the most popular of these products and is finally gaining the recognition it deserves. Long over-shadowed by another female hormone, estrogen, proges-terone also plays a major role in regulating the menstrual cycle. The sharp decline in production of both proges-terone and estrogen in midlife is what triggers menopause.

For decades, women have taken estrogen replacement therapy to treat the symptoms of menopause, such as hot flashes, insomnia, and depression. However, some women are reluctant to use estrogen because some studies suggest that it may increase the risk of breast cancer. Instead, these women have turned to natural progesterone creams, which offer many of the benefits of estrogen without the risk of cancer. Even better, natural progesterone actually protects against certain types of cancers, including uter-ine cancer. Progesterone is also a natural antidepressant and mood enhancer. In fact, it has been called the "feel-good" hormone for women because it can enhance libido and has a mild tranquilizing effect.

One of the primary reasons women take estrogen is to prevent osteoporosis, or the thinning of bone that can lead to fractures. After menopause, women lose 2 to 4 percent of bone mass each year annually for about ten years until the loss begins to level off, but by then much of the damage has already been done. Studies show that estrogen can reduce the risk of fractures by 50 percent, and many women believe that is good enough reason to bite the bullet and take it. There is good evidence, how-ever, that natural progesterone can halt the loss of bone as well as estrogen. According to animal studies per-formed by Dr. Jerilyn C. Prior of the University of British Columbia, natural progesterone not only can stop the loss of bone, like estrogen, but can stimulate osteoblasts, the cells that trigger the growth of new bone, which estrogen cannot do. Studies performed by Dr. John Lee, a

California physician who has written extensively on natural progesterone and prescribes it for his patients, confirm that progesterone can halt osteoporosis as effectively as estrogen.

Natural progesterone is not to be confused with progestins, which women take orally as part of hormone replacement therapy. Progestins are synthetic versions of progesterone but structurally different from the progesterone produced by a woman's body, and they often cause unpleasant side effects such as bloating, irritability, and mood swings. Natural progesterone is identical in chemical structure to the progesterone produced by the body.

POSSIBLE BENEFITS

Reduces common symptoms of menopause.
Prevents uterine cancer.
Stops the loss of bone that can lead to osteoporosis.

THE RIGHT AMOUNT

Use ¼ to ½ teaspoon of progesterone cream twice daily on abdomen, inner thighs, arms, or face.

Personal Advice

Find a natural healer or physician who can help you design your own natural menopause program based on your personal medical history and risk factors.

Neem (*Azadirachta indica*)

FACTS

This herb was hot 4,500 years ago, and it's hotter than ever today. Included in the ancient Indian Ayurvedic system of healing, neem is so versatile that it is known in

India as the "village pharmacy." Although neem has been used primarily in the treatment of skin diseases, inflammation, and fevers, there are more than 60 recorded uses for neem, ranging from insect repellent to skin cream to mouthwash. Recent studies have confirmed that neem is indeed powerful medicine.

Neem can be used externally, or internally as a dietary supplement. In India, neem paste is used to treat acne and eczema, a skin condition characterized by patchy red spots on the skin. In fact, neem is now being used in several different types of skin care products and is especially good for very dry, itchy, "winter skin." Even better, neem has natural antifungal, antiviral, and antibacterial properties, which means it can protect skin from common infections such as ringworm and scabies.

One of the most intriguing new uses for neem is as a toothpaste and mouthwash. For centuries, the bough of the neem plant was used in India as a makeshift toothbrush, and now researchers have discovered that neem's antibacterial and anti-inflammatory action is an effective treatment for gum disease. In particular, neem dental care products can help prevent the buildup of bacteria in the mouth that can lead to gum problems and tooth decay.

Neem is also an excellent natural insecticide and fertilizer. Insects do not eat leaves that have been sprayed with neem; if they do, they die. And unlike other insecticides that are harmful to humans, neem is actually beneficial. Neem products are sold at garden and lawn stores.

To add to its diversity, neem can also reduce fever when taken orally; it is similar in action to aspirin. I can just hear my doctor saying, "Take two neem and call me in the morning!"

POSSIBLE BENEFITS

Relieves eczema.
Is a natural moisturizer.
Helps prevent gum disease.
Is a natural insecticide.

THE RIGHT AMOUNT

Apply neem skin lotion to affected areas two or three times daily.
Use tooth and gum products as directed.

Olive Leaf Extract

FACTS

There is nothing new about olives and olive oil—both have been used for thousands of years for food. What is newsworthy, however, is olive leaf extract, an ancient treatment for a variety of ills that is being rediscovered by modern healers. As with so many other natural products, most of the scientific research on olive leaf extract has been performed in Europe. Unfortunately, there is often a time lag before this information filters down to the public, and olive leaf extract has only recently been introduced in the United States.

Olive leaf contains a biologically active compound, elenolic acid, which has strong antibacterial and antiviral properties. It disrupts the growth of bacteria and viruses and also stimulates the activity of important cells in the immune system that fight infection. In his intriguing new book *Olive Leaf Extract* (Nutriscreen, Inc., 1996), California physician James R. Privatera, M.D., describes his experience using olive leaf extract for patients with chronic viral or bacterial infections. Many of these patients had already received several courses of antibiotics, to no avail, but olive leaf extract was all it took to beat these infections. According to Dr. Privatera's findings, olive leaf extract is particularly effective against herpes, bladder, and fungal infections, which are often resistant to normal drug therapy. In particular, he reports excellent results in treating patients with *Candida albicans*, stubborn yeast infections. He also reports that several HIV-infected patients have seen improvement in immune function, notably a rise in disease-fighting T-cells, after taking olive leaf extract.

Olive leaf extract is also heart-friendly. Animal studies show that it can lower blood pressure and prevent the oxidation of LDL, or bad cholesterol, which can contribute to the formation of plaque that can clog arteries and cause heart disease. Since olive leaf extract behaves like an antioxidant, some researchers suspect that it may contain an antioxidant that has not yet been identified.

Olive leaf extract can be used by people who are suffering from chronic infections, especially those that have been resistant to other treatments.

POSSIBLE BENEFITS

Is effective against microbial infection.
Strengthens immune function.
Protects against heart disease.

THE RIGHT AMOUNT

For acute conditions (fevers, cold, flu, or fungal infections) take three 500-mg. tablets every four hours, or a total of 12 daily.
To prevent illness, take one 500-mg. tablet daily.

CAUTION

If a fever persists for more than a day, call your physician or natural healer.

Oregano Oil

FACTS

For thousands of years, oregano has been prized for its powerful antiseptic properties. The ancient Greeks used this herb to treat a wide variety of bacterial and viral infections. Today, oregano oil (available in liquid and capsules) is growing in popularity as an effective treatment for fungal infections, warts, psoriasis, eczema, viruses, and even the common cold.

First, let me clear up some common misconceptions about oregano. Dr. Cass Ingram explains in his book *The Cure Is in the Cupboard: How to Use Oregano for Better Health* that not everything called oregano is true oregano. Much of what passes for oregano is actually marjoram, which does not have the same healing properties as true oregano. To make sure you are getting the real thing, be sure to buy products that are derived from true oregano, known by the botanical name of *Origanum vulgare*.

Of the numerous compounds in oregano oil, the primary active ingredients are carvacrol and thymol, both potent antiseptics. In test tube studies, wild oregano has been shown to inhibit the growth of *Candida albicans*, the microbial cause of yeast infections. As I've already mentioned, oregano oil is also recommended for psoriasis and eczema, two skin conditions that can be aggravated by yeast infections.

Since oregano oil is an anti-inflammatory agent it can be rubbed on aching muscles to relieve strains, and used directly on minor burns and wounds to promote healing.

Long before pasteurization, bunches of oregano were hung in dairies to combat the proliferation of bacteria in milk. Today, we know that this practice was based on much more than mere superstition—it was good science. In one extraordinary Greek study, oregano oil showed strong antibacterial properties: even at dilutions as high as $\frac{1}{50,000}$, there was a significant decrease in bacterial growth.

Dr. Ingram writes about numerous patients who have benefited from oregano oil treatment for conditions ranging from flu to gum infections to cold sores to sports injuries. He cautions that a little oregano oil goes a long way, particularly if you ingest it.

POSSIBLE BENEFITS

Has natural antibiotic and antifungal properties.
Reduces inflammation.

THE RIGHT AMOUNT

For colds, flu, or Candida infection, take up to six capsules daily, as directed on the package, or 5 to 10 drops of oregano oil in liquid.

For warts and minor skin wounds, place a few drops of oregano oil on clean cotton swab and gently rub on the affected area. Use daily until healed.

Pepperine

FACTS

Pepperine is an extract derived from black pepper, a spice so highly prized for its flavor and medicinal properties that wars have been fought over it. Roman historians noted that Attila the Hun included 3,000 pounds of pepper as part of his ransom demands from the citizens of Rome. In fact, it was the search for pepper among other spices that ushered in the age of exploration and led to the discovery of the New World. Pepper owes its characteristic "hot" flavor to pepperine, a naturally occurring compound that can turn otherwise bland food into a taste sensation.

Pepperine is much more than a flavoring agent. It may play an important role in metabolism. Depending on how efficiently the body breaks down and utilizes food and supplements, nutrients are not always well absorbed. Because of a decrease in stomach acid and digestive enzymes, older people in particular have difficulty absorbing nutrients from supplements and food. In addition, compounds found in common foods, such as zinc, phytic acid in cereal, and caffeine in coffee, can block the absorption of vitamins and minerals. To complicate the problem, people on a low-fat diet may not be able to properly absorb fat-soluble vitamins such as vitamins A, E, and D. Studies have shown, however, that pepperine can enhance the absorption of nutrients so that more essential nutrients get to the tissues that need them. For example, in one study, healthy volunteers were given 5 mg. daily of a pepperine product (trademarked Bioperine) along with selected supplements, including beta carotene, selenium, and vitamin B_6. At the end of two weeks, blood levels of beta carotene increased by 60 percent over control subjects who were taking beta carotene alone. Within hours after they took pepperine, blood levels of selenium and vitamin B_6 were higher among pepperine users than nonusers. Although blood levels of these nutrients were increased, they were well within healthy, normal levels. None of the participants experienced any side effects.

Pepperine is sold in combination with other supplements, or in separate capsules.

POSSIBLE BENEFITS

Improves absorption of supplements.

THE RIGHT AMOUNT

Take three 5-mg. capsules daily.

CAUTION

If you are taking any medication, I don't recommend that you use pepperine, since there is a risk that it may result in higher-than-normal blood levels of the drug.

Phosphatidylcholine (PC)

FACTS

Phosphatidylcholine (PC), a naturally occurring phospholipid that is found in cell membranes, is the state-of-the-art supplement to reinvigorate a damaged liver. The liver is an incredibly hard-working organ that cleanses the blood of dangerous toxins from food, pollution, and chemical exposure. It also is vital for the metabolism of nutrients, produces clotting factors that promote wound healing, and is even involved in immune function.

Under the best of circumstances, the liver works amazingly hard, but some people force it to go into overdrive. For example, long-term exposure to drugs, pollutants, and excessive alcohol intake can compromise liver function. Alcohol, in particular, is a liver poison—heavy drinkers run the risk of developing cirrhosis of the liver, which can be fatal. In addition, commonly prescribed medicines such as cholesterol-lowering agents, chemotherapy drugs, and psychotropic drugs can cause liver damage over time, as can seemingly innocuous over-the-counter medications such as acetaminophen and aspirin. Infections like hepatitis, inflammation of the liver, can also result in impaired liver function. Numerous clinical studies have documented that PC can halt and even reverse liver damage, giving the liver time to heal. In particular, PC has been used on patients with hepatitis B infection and alcohol-related liver damage.

PC strengthens liver cell membranes, the gatekeepers that allow nutrients into the cells, but blocks damaging toxins from gaining entrance. PC also appears to stimulate cell regeneration, which helps to replace old, worn liver cells with youthful cells. Although PC is not a panacea—it won't cure every liver problem—it will help to speed up recovery for many people. PC is sold over the counter; however, if you have a history of liver problems or a current illness, you should be treated by a knowledgeable physician or healer who can help you to devise a program to promote liver health.

POSSIBLE BENEFITS

Supports liver function; helps to reverse damage.

THE RIGHT AMOUNT

Take six 230-mg. capsules daily. (Take three in the morning and three in the afternoon, with food.)

Phosphatidylserine (PS)

FACTS

Recently, a friend of mine in his 50s confessed that he was starting to forget things. It took him longer to recall phone numbers, he often forgot people's names, and if he didn't write something down he would forget to do it. Naturally, he was very worried about these changes. He was reassured to learn that everything he was describing was perfectly normal; in fact, there was even a name for his problem—age-associated memory impairment.

Once we reach our middle years, we begin to notice some subtle mental changes that are a direct result of aging. The most noticeable of these changes is a decline in short-term memory. While we can often remember things that occurred decades earlier in vivid detail, it is not unusual to forget someone's name the minute after we've been introduced. No one knows precisely why we experience midlife memory problems, but there is good evidence that they are caused by changes in brain chemistry. The brain contains a large amount of fatty tissue, including phospholipids, substances that not only hold cells together but control the entrance and exit of substances into the cells. Phosphatidylserine (PS) is one particularly important phospholipid that is involved in relaying chemical messages throughout the brain, helping brain cells to store and retrieve information. Once we reach middle age, phosphatidylserine and other important brain chemicals decline, which is one reason why our brains don't work as efficiently.

There is good evidence that taking phosphatidylserine supplements can help restore brain power. One recent study reported in the journal *Neurology* involved a group of 149 healthy men and women from 50 to 70 years of age who were diagnosed with normal age-associated memory problems. Participants were given 100 mg. of PS daily for 12 weeks, or a placebo. Those taking the PS noted significant improvements in their ability to recall telephone numbers, names, and faces; memorize paragraphs; find misplaced objects; and concentrate while performing tasks. Those who took the placebo showed virtually no change. In fact, according to the researcher who headed the study, PS supplements brought patients back an average of 12 years in their mental function! If you have age-related memory problems, I recommend that you give PS a try.

POSSIBLE BENEFITS

Enhances memory.
Improves your ability to concentrate.

THE RIGHT AMOUNT

Take up to two 300-mg. tablets daily.

Pregnenolone

FACTS

A supplement that can make you smarter and happier—and reduce the symptoms of arthritis? It sounds too good to be true, but if early studies pan out, pregnenolone may prove to be just that. Pregnenolone is a hormone produced by the brain and the adrenal glands, which sit above the kidneys. As we age, our levels of pregnenolone decline. At the same time, we also begin to experience age-related memory loss, particularly in short-term memory, and also have difficulty learning and memorizing new information.

Some researchers suspect that the decline in pregnenolone and related hormones may be responsible for memory problems experienced by older people, and they contend that boosting pregnenolone back to youthful levels could help restore memory and enhance learning. They point to early studies performed in the 1940s in which airline pilots were given pregnenolone to see if it could enhance concentration and job performance. Researchers trained 14 subjects to operate an airplane flight simulator machine that closely resembled the joysticks that are used on video games today. Before each session, the subjects were given either 50 mg. of pregnenolone or a placebo. Those taking pregnenolone showed improved concentration and a better ability to perform the task than those taking the placebo. In addition, the pilots said that they felt pregnenolone had helped them with actual flying, in that they fatigued less easily.

The same researchers tested pregnenolone on factory workers to see if it would have a positive effect on job performance. The workers taking pregnenolone not only were more productive but reported feeling happier and better able to cope with job-related stress. More recently, animal studies have shown that pregnenolone is one of the most potent memory-enhancing substances yet discovered, and that only a few molecules of it can dramatically improve memory in mice. Follow-up studies at St. Louis University showed that when given pregnenolone supplements three hours before testing, older men and women actually performed better on memory tests. When the results of these studies were reported in the press, pregnenolone became one of the most popular and hottest new supplements on the market.

Pregnenolone is gaining popularity as a treatment for rheumatoid arthritis (RA). In the 1940s, RA patients reported that pregnenolone helped to reduce the swelling, stiffness, and pain typical of their condition. It took about two weeks for pregnenolone to kick in, but once it did, patients were quite pleased with the result. Once cortisone was discovered in the late 1940s, however, interest in pregnenolone waned. Back then, cortisone seemed like a magic bullet that could eliminate arthritic symptoms practically overnight. What doctors didn't realize was that cortisone produced terrible side effects, including destruction of bone and a dampening effect on the immune system, which increased susceptibility to infection. More than 50 years later, there is still no cure for RA, and nearly every treatment brings with it substantial side effects. No wonder there is renewed interest in pregnenolone!

POSSIBLE BENEFITS

Improves concentration and memory.
Reduces stress.
May relieve symptoms of rheumatoid arthritis.

THE RIGHT AMOUNT

Take one 10-mg. tablet daily.

CAUTION

Because pregnenolone can elevate the levels of sex hormones, I recommend that you consult with a knowledgeable physician or natural healer before taking this hormone.

Proanthocyanidins (PCOs)

FACTS

Proanthocyanidins (PCOs) are antioxidants found in the bark, stems, leaves, and skins of some plants. In 1947, PCOs were first isolated from the red inner skin of the peanut by French research scientist Dr. Jack Masquelier. Today, PCOs are derived from grapeseed and pine bark extract. Although they occur naturally in fruits and vegetables, PCOs are often discarded in normal food handling and cooking. This is unfortunate, because they offer some truly wonderful health benefits. PCOs are powerful vascular protectors that support the body's circulatory system, the vast network of capillaries, arteries, and veins that keep blood flowing to the cells where it is needed. PCOs help maintain good circulation by blocking the formation of cholesterol deposits on artery walls. In France, where natural remedies are more readily accepted than in the United States, PCOs are widely used to treat high cholesterol and prevent heart disease. PCOs are also used to treat problems of venous insufficiency, or poor circulation, which can cause nerve damage or blood clots in the legs.

PCOs also have a protective effect on collagen, the cellular glue that holds skin and other structures together. Collagen, the primary protein found in connective tissue, is especially vulnerable to free radical attack. PCOs inhibit the activity of harmful enzymes that, if allowed to attack collagen, can weaken and destroy it. In fact, many changes in the body we associate with normal aging are actually caused by free radical damage. For example, if the collagen on an artery wall is damaged, it can make the arteries rigid and promote the buildup of plaque, which can lead to clot formation. If a clot forms in the artery delivering blood to the heart, it can trigger a heart attack; if it forms in the artery delivering blood to the brain, it can result in a stroke. Collagen is also essential for maintaining healthy bones, cartilage, gums, and eyes.

In their role as a collagen protector, PCOs are not only critical for good health but can also help you look good. PCOs may prevent skin from aging by protecting collagen from free radical damage, which can cause skin to sag and promote the formation of wrinkles.

PCOs are also powerful chelating agents; that is, they can protect the body from unstable metals that can promote oxidative damage and contribute to free radical damage. PCOs can be purchased as a single supplement or in combination formulas designed to enhance cardiovascular health.

POSSIBLE BENEFITS

Promotes good circulation.
Protects collagen from free radical damage.

THE RIGHT AMOUNT

Take up to three 30- to 100-mg. tablets daily between meals. People who are older or who have compromised immune systems may need the higher dose. Healthier young people can try the lower dose.

Probiotics

FACTS

Since the discovery of the first antibiotic, penicillin, these drugs have been our primary weapons in the war against disease. Unfortunately, the overuse of antibiotics has led to the rise of drug-resistant bacteria and, consequently, infections that can be lethal. In addition, antibiotics are useless against viral infections such as HIV infection and hepatitis. That is why a growing number of physicians and natural healers are taking a probiotic approach to keeping their patients well.

Probiotic, which means "for life," is a general term for microorganisms also known as friendly bacteria, which bolster the body's own defenses against disease. Our bodies are host to several thousand billion friendly bacteria—more than all the cells in your body. These bacteria play a role in digestion and also work in tandem with our immune system to keep us healthy. Among their many jobs, friendly bacteria manufacture some B vitamins, help normalize hormone levels, can help reduce cholesterol levels, and protect against pollutants. They also play a major role in immune function. As we age, we experience a drop in these good bacteria, which makes us more vulnerable to disease. Therefore, it is imperative to restore friendly bacteria back to youthful levels by taking probiotic supplements.

The most beneficial of the friendly bacteria are *Bifidobacterium*, *Lactobacillus acidophilus*, and *Lactobacillus bulgaricus*. One of the most important roles of friendly bacteria is to protect us from overgrowth and infection from fungi and yeasts, which can produce toxic and carcinogenic substances. If left unchecked they may be absorbed into the bloodstream and contribute to other diseases. The most exciting research on good bacteria is their role in supporting the immune system. Bifidobacteria, in particular, have inhibitory effects on pathogens such as *Salmonella*, *Staphylococcus aureus*, and *Candida albicans*. In addition, bifidobacteria also have anticarcinogenic and tumor suppressing effects.

One reason I try to avoid taking antibiotics is that these drugs cannot distinguish between good and bad bacteria—they kill whatever crosses their path. Corticosteroids and birth control pills can also kill friendly bacteria.

So, how do we increase our levels of good bacteria? Eating the right foods can help. A fiber-rich diet can help because intestinal bacteria consume dietary fiber and metabolize it into organic acids that inhibit the growth of bad bacteria. Nonfat or low-fat yogurt made with live, active cultures is another immune-boosting food that is a rich source of friendly bacteria.

The easiest way to ensure that you have enough friendly bacteria on hand is to take a daily probiotic supplement, which is sold at health food stores. These supplements come in capsules, liquids, or powders. In fact, probiotics are so popular that some natural food stores have an entire section devoted to them.

POSSIBLE BENEFITS

Can enhance immune function.
Helps control yeast infections.
May protect against cancer.

THE RIGHT AMOUNT

Take three capsules (containing billions of organisms) daily, half an hour before meals.
Take 1 tablespoon of liquid half an hour before meals.

Personal Advice

If you must use an antibiotic, it is especially important to take probiotic supplements during the time you are taking the drug and for as long as a month afterward to replenish the healthful bacteria that may be killed along with the bad bacteria.

When you first start taking probiotics, you may notice an increase in gassiness or bloating, which is a sign that the good bacteria are fermenting. Within a week or two, your body will adjust to the change.

Puncturevine (*Tribulus terrestis*)

FACTS

Puncturevine, also called tribulus after its botanical name, is the talk of the town. Growing in popularity by leaps and bounds, this "new" supplement has actually been around more than 5,000 years as part of the traditional healing systems of China and India. Why is it so hot today? Tribulus has special appeal to men because it promises to boost their performance in two key areas: the gym and the bedroom.

The buzz among body builders is that tribulus can stimulate the production of testosterone, which will help build muscle and burn fat. Their assertions are based on Bulgarian studies that showed that tribulus naturally increased the body's production of luteinizing hormone (LH), which stimulates the production of testosterone in men and estrogen in women. In fact, in Eastern Europe, both male and female Olympic athletes reportedly use tribulus to give them a competitive edge. Unlike anabolic steroids, which are banned from most competitions, there are no rules against tribulus.

Claims that tribulus will enhance sexual performance in men can also be traced to Bulgarian studies in which athletes who took tribulus claimed that it increased their sex drive and performance. In addition, tribulus is reputed to increase fertility and sperm production. There are many anecdotal reports to back up this claim, but I was not able to find any clinical studies specifically related to sexual problems.

Since it may also boost estrogen levels in women, tribulus is being promoted as a treatment for menopausal symptoms such as hot flashes and fatigue.

Tribulus supplements often include natural hormones such as DHEA and androstenedione, a metabolite of DHEA. Since tribulus may raise testosterone levels, men who have a history of prostate cancer should steer clear of this supplement.

POSSIBLE BENEFITS

Builds muscle.
Improves sexual performance.

THE RIGHT AMOUNT

Take up to two 125-mg. tablets on an empty stomach with a full glass of water.

Pygeum (*Pygeum africanum*)

FACTS

As the American population ages and baby boomer men turn 50, I am constantly asked about natural remedies to prevent or treat common prostate problems. For general prostate health, I often recommend pygeum, an herb that is derived from the bark of the African evergreen.

The prostate gland is a small, walnut-sized gland located above the rectum. As men age, the prostate becomes enlarged, resulting in a condition known as benign prostate hypertrophy (BPH). If the prostate becomes very swollen, it can press against the urethra and interfere with urination. Difficult urination and frequent urination, especially at night, are the most common symptoms of BPH. In about 10 percent of all men, BPH will become so severe that they will require corrective surgery.

Pygeum combined with another herb, saw palmetto

(see page 154), not only is a very effective treatment for BPH but, I believe, can help prevent early symptoms from becoming more serious. I take a combination of herbs, including pygeum, saw palmetto, and stinging nettle, to prevent prostate problems from occurring at all. Men who have suffered from severe BPH symptoms report that pygeum can help reduce nighttime urination and the interruption of urinary flow.

Pygeum is also reputed to be an aphrodisiac, and at least one study has shown that men who took pygeum for BPH reported an increase in sexual activity. In fact, one Italian researcher noted that among patients with BPH, pygeum treatment actually improved their ability to achieve an erection. Of course, the renewed interest in sex could be due to the fact that these men were no longer preoccupied with their prostate woes and were well enough to feel romantic!

POSSIBLE BENEFITS

Reduces symptoms of BPH.

THE RIGHT AMOUNT

Take up to three 500-mg. capsules daily with a full glass of water.

Pyruvate

FACTS

Lose weight and burn fat without lifting a finger? It may sound too good to be true, but studies suggest that pyruvate may actually reduce body fat and increase muscle tone *without* exercise. Even better, this new sports supplement can also help you lose weight. In one study conducted at the University of Pittsburgh, obese women were given a low-fat diet and then given either pyruvate supplements or a placebo. After three weeks, the women taking pyruvate had lost 37 percent more weight and nearly 50 percent more fat than the women taking the placebo. And unlike prescription diet drugs that have recently been shown to cause heart problems, pyruvate is actually good for your heart: It can lower blood cholesterol levels and blood pressure, thereby reducing the risk of heart disease.

Pyruvate is naturally found in the body as a by-product of normal metabolism. It is critical for energy use because it triggers the release of ATP, the fuel produced by the cells that provides energy for the entire body.

In another recent study, athletes who used pyruvate tired less easily and were able to increase their performance by an impressive 20 percent.

If you use pyruvate you are in good company. Many well-known athletes and fitness mavens swear by pyruvate, including the Green Bay Packers as well as Shannon Miller, gold medalist in the 1996 Olympic games.

POSSIBLE BENEFITS

Burns fat.
Promotes weight loss.
Increases energy and stamina.
Improves cardiovascular health.

THE RIGHT AMOUNT

As a sports supplement, take six to eight 500-mg. tablets daily before exercise or a meal.
For weight loss, take at least 4 grams (4000 mg.) per day.

Quercetin

FACTS

Closely related to rutin (see page 149) and hesperidin, quercetin is fast becoming a superstar among the bioflavonoids. Discovered in the 1930s by Nobel Prize laureate Albert Szent-Gzorgy, who called them vitamin P, bioflavonoids have had a rocky history. Szent-Gzorgy reported that these substances could strengthen capillaries (tiny blood vessels) and improve circulation. At one time, physicians prescribed bioflavonoids for bleeding gums and circulatory problems. In 1968, for reasons that now seem nothing less than lunatic, the FDA deemed bioflavonoids to be worthless. Thanks to the work of a few persistent researchers, close to 30 years later, we now know that these substances are worth their weight in gold.

Many flavonoids, including quercetin, are potent cancer fighters. Found in red and yellow onions, grapes, and Italian squash, quercetin is now believed to be one of the most powerful anticancer substances discovered to date. According to a recent study published by the National Cancer Institute and the Beijing Institute for Cancer Research, people who ate the most quercetin-rich onions (and garlic, which does not contain quercetin but is rich in beneficial sulfur compounds) had a 20-fold lower cancer risk than people who did not. Furthermore, test tube and animal studies have documented that quercetin stops cancer at its earliest stage by preventing the damaging changes in the cells that initiate cancer, and thwarting the spread of cancer cells.

Recently, quercetin has attracted attention as an effective treatment for allergies and inflammatory disorders. Quercetin blocks the release of histamines, proteins that cause the sneezing, stuffy nose, watery eyes, and other symptoms characteristic of an allergic reaction. In fact, quercetin is similar to the prescription antiallergy drug cromolyn sodium, which also prevents the release of histamines. Along with other bioflavonoids, quercetin is typically included in allergy relief combination formulas sold at natural food stores. In addition, quercetin can block the release of even stronger inflammatory agents, leukotrienes, which are involved in asthma, psoriasis, gout, ulcerative colitis, and other common ailments. Although everyone can benefit from quercetin, people with allergies and inflammatory conditions should be vigilant about getting enough of this bioflavonoid. If you don't eat an onion or two daily, take quercetin supplements.

POSSIBLE BENEFITS

Strengthens capillaries, promotes good circulation.
Is a powerful anticancer compound.
Is a natural anti-inflammatory agent.
Can relieve allergic symptoms.

THE RIGHT AMOUNT

Take one 400-mg. capsule before each meal.

Red Wine Polyphenols

FACTS

It's been called the French Paradox. Even though they gorge on cheese and goose liver pâté, drench their food in cream sauce, eat other high-fat foods with abandon, and smoke like chimneys, the French have one of the lowest rates of heart disease in the world. Some researchers

suspect that the French may owe their good health to the
way they typically wash down their meals with a glass or
two of wine. Wine, particularly red wine, is a rich source
of polyphenols, potent antioxidants that protect against
heart disease by blocking the oxidation of LDL, the bad
cholesterol. When LDL becomes oxidized, or rancid, it
can promote the formation of plaque in arterial walls,
which blocks the flow of blood and oxygen. Numerous
studies have shown that red wine polyphenols can slow
down blood clotting, which is important because blood
clots are a major cause of heart attack and stroke.

There's even more good news about red wine polyphenols. Recently, researchers at the University of California
at Davis reported that red wine polyphenols slowed the
formation of tumors in mice bred to develop the types of
cancers that afflict humans.

Despite all these wonderful discoveries about red wine
polyphenols, there is a downside to drinking wine, at
least every day. First, wine is fattening: one 4-ounce glass
contains 100 calories. If you have two glasses of wine
every day, you have added 1400 additional calories each
week, which adds up to ten unwanted pounds each year.
Second, red wine can give some people headaches, especially those who are prone to migraine. Third, excess
alcohol can cause serious liver damage. Last, and most
important, many people have problems with alcohol
addiction, and wine is off limits for them. But these problems don't mean you have to forgo the benefits of wine.
The same polyphenols found in red wine are now available in capsules. For those who don't want to drink (or
who may drink wine only occasionally, as I do), it is a
terrific way to have your polyphenols without the excess
calories or the hangover.

POSSIBLE BENEFITS

May help prevent heart disease by its antioxidant action.
May protect against cancer.

THE RIGHT AMOUNT

Take two 30-mg. capsules daily.

Resveratrol

FACTS

In my book *Earl Mindell's Food as Medicine*, I wrote about special compounds found in grapes that protect against disease. At the time that book was written, Japanese researchers had just discovered an antifungal compound in grapes called resveratrol, which lowered cholesterol levels in rats and showed promise of doing the same in humans. Since then, researchers at the University of Illinois, under the direction of Dr. John Pezzuto, have uncovered new and exciting information about resveratrol. Studies have shown that resveratrol may prevent heart disease in two important ways. First, it inhibits the formation of blood clots, which can trigger both heart attack and stroke. Second, it plays a role in cholesterol metabolism, which may prevent the formation of artery-clogging plaque.

What's even more exciting, however, is resveratrol's potential as cancer fighter. In one study, mice bred to develop skin cancer were given resveratrol supplements. At the end of 18 weeks, the mice given resveratrol had 98 percent fewer skin tumors than those who had not been given the supplement. In studies of human leukemia cells, resveratrol inhibited the formation of abnormal cells; even more importantly, it was able to turn malignant cells back to normal.

Until recently, the only way to obtain the benefits of resveratrol was to drink wine or grape juice. For the first time, resveratrol is now available in supplement form.

POSSIBLE BENEFITS

Reduces the risk of heart disease.
Inhibits the formation of cancerous tumors.

THE RIGHT AMOUNT

Take one 1000-mcg. capsule daily.

Rosemary (*Rosmarinus officinalis*)

FACTS

For centuries, rosemary has been known as the herb for remembrance, but it soon may also become equally well known as the herb that fights cancer. The Rosemary Study, a fascinating research project conducted at Penn State and reported in the May 1996 *Journal of Nutrition*, revealed that rosemary could significantly reduce the risk of cancer in rats given a powerful carcinogen. In one experiment, researchers fed laboratory rats a diet supplemented with 1 percent rosemary for two weeks, using the same dried rosemary leaves available at supermarkets. Then, the rosemary-fed rats were given a known carcinogen that binds to breast cells and can damage DNA, thereby promoting cancer. The study showed that the cancer-causing chemical was much less likely to bind to breast cells in the rats fed rosemary than in those that were not, which strongly suggests that rosemary can inhibit the early stages of tumor formation.

There is new scientific evidence to confirm rosemary's long-held reputation as a memory enhancer. Studies show that rosemary contains acetylcholinesterase inhibitors, substances that can block the breakdown of acetylcholine, a neurotransmitter involved in mental function. Low levels of acetylcholine have been associated with normal age-related memory loss and with Alzheimer's disease. Studies of Alzheimer's patients are under way to determine if using rosemary oil in bath water or directly on the skin can slow down or even stop the progression of this disease.

POSSIBLE BENEFITS

May prevent normal cells from turning cancerous.
Can help prevent memory loss.

THE RIGHT AMOUNT

Take up to two 500-mg. capsules daily.

Royal Jelly

FACTS

It's interesting that two of the Hot 100 supplements are products that are either used or made by bees and have been around for about 40 million years! Bee propolis, also known as bee glue, made from plants and other substances and used by bees to seal and disinfect the hive, is described on page 7. Royal jelly is a white, milky secretion produced by worker bees, the hard-working insects that keep the beehive humming with activity. During the first three days of life, all bee larvae eat this special foodstuff, but after that, the only bee that continues to eat the royal jelly is the designated queen bee. The queen bee grows to be 50 percent larger than the other female bees in the hive, lives up to 40 times longer, and is highly fertile, compared with the sterile worker bees. Herbalists have long believed that the royal jelly is what gives the queen bee her obvious advantage over other bees.

Royal jelly is a complete protein, containing all essential amino acids and B vitamins. Studies have shown that royal jelly is a mild antibiotic and has a stimulating effect on the adrenal glands, which produce key hormones in the body that regulate metabolism, mood, appetite, and even sex drive. Herbalists often recommend royal jelly for menopause problems in women, to improve sexual performance in men, and as an energizing tonic for both sexes. Anecdotal evidence suggests that royal jelly may help reduce the appearance of fine lines and wrinkles. If royal jelly works as well on humans as it does on queen bees, it may help us live longer, healthier lives.

POSSIBLE BENEFITS

Increases energy, restores sex drive.
Improves quality of skin.
Helps treat symptoms of menopause.

THE RIGHT AMOUNT

Take up to two 500-mg. capsules daily.

Personal Advice

I take two capsules daily to boost energy and stamina.

Rutin

FACTS

Rutin is one of several bioflavonoids that provide color and taste to fruits and vegetables and do much, much more. Bioflavonoids are meant to work together, and not surprisingly, rutin supplements often include other bioflavonoids such as quercetin and hesperidin. Bioflavonoids in general, and rutin in particular, can strengthen capillaries, the tiniest blood vessels. Rutin is essential for the proper absorption and use of vitamin C and assists vitamin C in maintaining collagen, the tissue beneath the skin that supports the epidermis, the outer layer of cells.

The most popular use for rutin is as a treatment for allergies. Studies show that rutin can slow down the release of histamine, the chemical released by mast cells that trigger common allergic reactions such as a stuffy nose. In fact, rutin is typically included in special anti-allergy formulas designed to relieve the symptoms of hay fever and asthma. Most people find that these preparations are very effective and do not cause the side effects, such as drowsiness or dry mouth, that are typical of many antihistamine medications.

Because of its ability to strengthen capillaries, rutin may also be an effective treatment for bruises, varicose veins (caused by a weakness in the blood vessels), and hemorrhoids, an inflammation of the veins in the anus and rectum. Like other flavonoids, rutin is an anti-inflammatory agent, and also shows antiviral, antimicrobial, and anticancer activity. I have no doubt that the more we study rutin, the more uses we will find for it.

POSSIBLE BENEFITS

Relieves allergy.
Helps reduce black-and-blue bruise marks on skin.

THE RIGHT AMOUNT

Take up to three 100- to 500-mg. tablets daily, at least half
an hour before meals.

S-Adenosyl-L-Methione (SAMe)

FACTS

In recent years, researchers have focused on changes within the body that may set the stage for the downward spiral we have long associated with normal aging. The age-related decline in the production of key hormones such as estrogen, DHEA, and testosterone has received a great deal of attention lately. So has the age-related decline in important antioxidants produced by the body to defend against free radicals. To compensate for these losses, many people take supplemental hormones and antioxidants to restore them back to their youthful protective levels. Now, a growing number of researchers say there is yet another group of compounds we need to replenish as we age: methyl groups.

Methyl groups promote methylation, a process whereby homocysteine, a potentially dangerous amino acid, is converted into methionine, a beneficial compound. At any age, high blood levels of homocysteine have been associated with an increased risk of heart disease, cancer, depression, arthritis, birth defects, and other diseases. Only a handful of compounds can promote methylation, including the B vitamins folic acid and vitamin B_{12}, and trimethylglycine (TMG) (see page 168). One of the beneficial byproducts of methylation is an increase in the levels of SAMe, a metabolite of methionine that also declines with age. SAMe is essential for the synthesis of melatonin, the antiaging hormone that regulates the sleep/wake cycles (see page 107). It also helps to protect DNA from mutations that could promote cancer, prevents peripheral nerve damage due to lack of oxygen, and may play a role in deactivating harmful homocysteine.

As if this were not enough to earn SAMe a place on the Hot 100, SAMe is also reputed to be a highly effective antidepressant that works as well as many prescription drugs but without the unpleasant and potentially dangerous side effects. In one study published in the *American Journal of Psychiatry*, 15 patients suffering from major depression were treated with SAMe for three weeks and experienced a 50 percent improvement according to usual psychiatric evaluation procedures.

SAMe is also gaining fame as an excellent treatment for the aches and pains associated with osteoarthritis, and it is as effective an anti-inflammatory agent as ibuprofen. In a two-year German study, 108 patients with osteoporosis of the knee, hip, and spine were given 600 mg. of SAMe daily. By the second week of treatment, researchers noted improvement in joint pain, notably in morning stiffness and pain on rest and moving. A small number of patients experienced only minor side effects, none serious enough to warrant discontinuation of treatment. Other European studies suggest that SAMe may help control the joint pain and depression associated with fibromyalgia, a mysterious disorder characterized by unspecified aches, pains, and fatigue. Since there is no cure for fibromyalgia, many patients have turned to natural remedies, including coenzyme-Q10, and grapeseed and green tea extracts in combination tablets. If you have fibromyalgia, talk to your physician about using SAMe.

POSSIBLE BENEFITS

Works as a natural antidepressant.
May control the joint pain typical of arthritic type syndromes.
May help treat dementia in elderly people.

THE RIGHT AMOUNT

Take up to three 500-mg. capsules daily.

Saint John's Wort (*Hypericum performatum*)

FACTS

Undoubtedly you have seen the signs in natural food stores and pharmacies proclaiming in big letters, "We have Saint John's wort." Saint John's wort has become one of the most popular of all herbal supplements and has received much positive attention from the media in recent months. Why all the excitement?

A longtime folk remedy for the treatment of mild depression, Saint John's wort has gotten the stamp of approval from the medical establishment. Recently, an article in the prestigious *British Medical Journal* reviewed 30 separate studies on this herb and concluded that it is as effective an antidepressant as any prescription drug. In nearly every study, patients taking Saint John's wort reported a decrease in feelings of depression and an improvement in mood, but without any of the unpleasant side effects typical of prescription drugs such as dry mouth, constipation, and dizziness.

Another advantage of Saint John's wort over prescription medication is that it costs only pennies a day as opposed to several dollars a day. Europeans have been using Saint John's wort for decades; it is the leading antidepressant in Germany. In the United States, however, where our health care system is dominated by the pharmaceutical industry, physicians usually prescribe the antidepressant *du jour*. The word on Saint John's wort is so good that the National Institutes of Health will soon sponsor double-blind clinical trials of this herb.

Saint John's wort is nature's cure for depression, but is it also a cure for obesity? A new product called "herbal Phen Fen" is being sold at natural food stores and pharmacies. "Herbal Phen Fen" contains Saint John's wort and ephedra, an herb that is used in antihistamines but that can also increase metabolism. Very preliminary studies suggest that Saint John's wort can help control appetite and food cravings and, when combined with ephedra, will produce dramatic weight loss. Because of the recent withdrawal of real Phen-Fen, an herbal alternative may be just what the doctor ordered. Although these products may be safe and effective, there are few studies to confirm this. If used in excess, ephedra can cause dangerous side effects such as heart arrhythmia. Therefore, if you use "herbal Phen-Fen," be *sure* to follow the directions carefully and do not exceed the recommended dose. I advise that anyone who has a history of heart disease, or who is taking a prescription antidepressant, first obtain medical advice from a doctor or natural healer before taking this preparation.

The unusual name of Saint John's wort dates back to the Middle Ages. Legend has it that this plant sprang from Saint John the Baptist's blood when he was beheaded.

POSSIBLE BENEFITS

Relieves depression.
May help to control appetite.

THE RIGHT AMOUNT

Take up to three 250- to 500-mg. capsules daily.

CAUTION

Saint John's wort can increase sensitivity to the sun. Therefore, be sure to wear sunscreen and avoid direct exposure.

Saw Palmetto

FACTS

Calling all guys over 50—this supplement is for you! Saw palmetto is *the* herb for prostate health, an issue that should concern all middle-aged men. The prostate is a small, walnut-shaped gland that surrounds the part of the urethra located under the bladder. At about age 40, hormonal changes can begin to cause problems for the prostate. Levels of the hormone prolactin rise, stimulating the production of the enzyme 5-alpha reductase, which in turn converts testosterone into a more potent form called dihydrotestosterone. Dihydrotestosterone can trigger the growth of prostate tissue, which results in a condition known as benign prostate hypertrophy (BPH).

Although it is not life-threatening, BPH can be a real nuisance and can cause unpleasant symptoms such as the need to urinate frequently, especially at night, and difficulty passing urine, which can be extremely frustrating. Standard drug therapy for BPH can cause some equally unpleasant symptoms, such as loss of libido, dizziness, and even depression.

The good news is that saw palmetto can help keep BPH under control so that in most cases drugs are not necessary. First used by Native Americans to treat prostate problems and urinary tract infections, saw palmetto has been shown by more than 20 studies to help relieve the common symptoms of BPH. How? Saw palmetto gets to the root of the problem by controlling the hormonal changes that stimulate prostatic growth. I recommend saw palmetto for men who already have BPH and for those who want to avoid it.

Since BPH is so very common among middle-aged men, it is not surprising that dozens of new prostate products containing saw palmetto as well as other herbs, vitamins, and minerals have appeared on the shelves of health food stores. Look for products that include, in addition to saw palmetto, stinging nettles (a wonderful natural diuretic), the mineral zinc, which is found in high concentration in the prostate, and pygeum (see page 139), another herb that can relieve the symptoms of BPH.

POSSIBLE BENEFITS

Relieves the symptoms of BPH.
Maintains the health of the prostate.

THE RIGHT AMOUNT

Take up to three 500-mg. capsules daily.

Sea Cucumber

FACTS

Sea cucumbers are so low on the evolutionary scale that it's hard to tell whether they are flora or fauna. Despite their name and plantlike appearance, sea cucumbers are living, breathing creatures that inhabit the oceans of the world.

For centuries, sea cucumbers have been used in Asia for food and for medicinal purposes. Recently, a supplement made from home-grown sea cucumber caught off the coast of Maine has become a popular treatment for arthritis. According to Pete Collin of Coastside Bio Resources in Stonington, Maine, the body walls of sea cucumber are similar to human cartilage. Sea cucumber is an excellent source of glucosamine (see page 63) and chondroitin sulfate (see page 27), which are important building blocks of cartilage, the connective tissue that absorbs shock and protects bones. It is the wearing down of cartilage that causes bones to rub together, triggering the pain and inflammation typical of arthritis.

In addition to these two substances, sea cucumber contains another recently discovered substance that according to laboratory reports is an even more potent anti-inflammatory agent than hydrocortisone. Although hydrocortisone is a wonderful anti-inflammatory agent and pain reliever, it can produce serious side effects. Notably, hydrocortisone can raise blood pressure, increase cholesterol, weaken bones, thin the skin, and depress immune function. Numerous anecdotal reports confirm that sea cucumber can reduce the pain and stiffness associated with arthritic diseases, bursitis, and other problems of the bones and joints without any of the problems associated with hydrocortisone. Athletes also use sea cucumber to promote healing of cartilage injuries, which can occur as part of the normal wear and tear of an active lifestyle.

Arthritis afflicts not only humans but older animals as well. Sea cucumber is also an effective treatment for animals suffering from the aches and pains of arthritis.

POSSIBLE BENEFITS

Relieves symptoms of arthritis.
Promotes healing of athletic injuries.

THE RIGHT AMOUNT

Take up to six 600-mg. capsules daily with meals.

Shark Liver Oil

FACTS

The best-selling book *Sharks Don't Get Cancer* introduced shark cartilage as a potential treatment for many different types of cancer. Shark cartilage works by inhibiting the process of angiogenesis, whereby new blood vessels are formed to deliver blood and nutrients to the tumor. If the tumor is denied blood, it cannot grow, and the cancer cannot spread. Researchers are now saying that a different part of the shark—the liver—may be an even more potent cancer fighter than the cartilage.

Shark liver oil is rich in vitamins A and D and also contains the biologically active compounds squalene and alkyglycerol (AKG), which are being studied for their disease-fighting properties. In addition, it contains other substances that may prove to be important for health. The net effect is that shark liver oil has a remarkable effect on the immune system. It enhances the production of macrophages, a type of white blood cell that helps control viral and yeast infections. And numerous studies have documented the ability of shark liver oil to inhibit chemically induced cancers in animals.

Shark liver oil can also protect against radiation injury, which may benefit cancer patients. Exposure to radiation normally results in depressed immune function, which includes a reduction in disease-fighting white cells and lymphocytes. However, when squalene, a component of shark liver oil, was added to their diet, animals exposed to a lethal dose of radiation maintained stronger immune systems and lived significantly longer than animals that were not given shark liver oil. Because of the positive results of these animal studies, shark liver oil is now being investigated as a cancer treatment for humans in combination with other therapies. Studies in Europe and Japan have shown that giving cancer patients shark liver oil before, during, and after radiation treatment will also help reduce some of the negative effects on immune function that often occur after treatment.

In addition to bolstering immune function, shark liver oil is a strong antioxidant that can protect cell membranes from free radical attack. If free radicals are allowed to penetrate the cell membranes, they can cause permanent damage that can lead to cancer and other diseases. Shark liver oil supplements are taken daily to enhance immune function and to fortify against colds and other infections.

There are several shark liver oil products on the market of varying quality. The best products clearly list their squalene and AKG content; some researchers believe that sharks that live in deep, cold water are the richest source of these unique compounds. In addition, look for minimally processed oils—the more processing, the more likely it is that beneficial ingredients are destroyed.

POSSIBLE BENEFITS

Strengthens immune function.
May thwart the growth of cancerous cells.

THE RIGHT AMOUNT

Take one capsule or 1 teaspoon of oil daily.

Silicon (Silica)

FACTS

The word *silicon* may conjure up images of computer chips, but you may not know that this mineral is also essential for your body. Natural healers have long recommended horsetail, an herb rich in silicon, to help restore dull, lifeless hair and chipped, dry nails. Silicon (sometimes called silica) is now being marketed as a supplement in its own right. (The mineral silicon is not to be confused with the compound silicone, the material in breast implants.)

Silicon is important for the maintenance of bones; connective tissue, as in the tendons that connect bones to joints; and collagen, the underlying structure that holds skin in place. Silicon can also help keep blood vessels healthy by preserving their elasticity and strength, thereby enhancing blood flow throughout the body. Many athletes and body builders take silicon supplements to help prevent connective tissue injury and to speed up recovery if they are already injured.

Although there is no scientific evidence to back this claim, some natural healers prescribe silicon to forestall hair loss. Since silicon helps in the absorption of calcium, it is also being investigated as a treatment for osteoporosis. Silicon levels decrease with age, and some researchers believe the decline in this mineral may promote connective tissue problems as well as wrinkled skin. There are anecdotal reports that silicon can cure common nail problems, such as peeling and white spots. Some studies have shown that silicon can also enhance immune function and, in particular, can increase the level of immune cells that weed out toxins and infections.

POSSIBLE BENEFITS

Enhances calcium absorption, strengthens bones.
Protects connective tissue.
Improves hair and nails.

THE RIGHT AMOUNT

Take up to three 500-mg. capsules or tablets up to three times daily.

Silymarin

FACTS

Silymarin is a supplement that contains three bioflavonoids extracted from the milk thistle plant: silybin, silydianin, and silychristin. Since ancient times, milk thistle has been the primary herb used to treat liver disorders. Modern scientific research has confirmed that silymarin does indeed enhance liver function.

One of the hardest-working organs in the body, the liver detoxifies the poisons that enter our bloodstream, including nicotine, alcohol, chemicals, drugs, and pollutants. Exposure to chemicals, infections, or poisons can promote the formation of free radicals, which can cause oxidative damage to liver cells. Silymarin is an antioxidant that can not only block the destructive action of free radicals but also increase the levels of glutathione and superoxide dismutase, two of the body's own most important antioxidants.

Silymarin can also help repair damaged or injured liver cells. Natural healers use silymarin to treat many liver problems, including damage due to excess alcohol consumption, jaundice, hepatitis, and even amanita mushroom poisoning, which can be lethal. In animal studies, when silymarin is given within 24 hours of amanita mushroom consumption, it can help prevent serious liver damage that can lead to death.

There have also been numerous human clinical studies performed on silymarin, primarily in Europe. Some of the most successful have involved patients suffering from cirrhosis of the liver due to alcohol damage. In one study, patients suffering from cirrhosis of the liver who were given silymarin lived longer than those who were given a placebo. German scientists are now evaluating the use of silymarin on patients with viral hepatitis along with other medications. Earlier studies have been quite promising and show that silymarin can help improve common symptoms such as fatigue, loss of appetite, and abdominal discomfort.

The eclectic physicians, herbal healers from the turn of the century, used milk thistle to treat psoriasis, a skin condition that may be aggravated by sluggish liver function, which allows toxins to form in the blood.

Don't get the idea, however, that silymarin is just for people with specific liver disorders. I believe it can be particularly useful for people who are exposed to toxins on the job, such as people who work near chemical plants or beauty parlors, or who live in polluted areas.

POSSIBLE BENEFITS

Protects liver from free radical damage.

May be a useful treatment for hepatitis and cirrhosis of the liver.

May improve overall liver function.

THE RIGHT AMOUNT

Take up to three 500-mg. tablets or capsules daily.

Soy Concentrate (Isolates)

FACTS

Recently I watched a special report on the nightly news about a major medical breakthrough. According to a recent study, a diet rich in soy foods may reduce the risk of breast cancer and possibly even prostate cancer. I thought to myself, "Hey guys, where have you been? I've been saying this for years!" In fact, you can read all about it in my book *Earl Mindell's Soy Miracle* (Fireside, 1995), where I sing the praises of soy as a potent cancer fighter. In Japan and other countries where people regularly eat soy food, such as soy milk, tofu, miso, and tempeh, the risk of dying of either breast or prostate cancer is minuscule compared with countries like the United States where soy is not a dietary staple.

On average, the Japanese eat 3 to 4 ounces of soy food daily; Americans typically eat none. Sadly, American women are four times more likely to die of breast cancer than are Japanese women, and American men are five times more likely to die of prostate cancer than are Japanese men. At one time it was believed that the difference in cancer rates between the two countries was simply genetics, but that didn't explain why, when Japanese emigrated to the United States, within one generation they had the same cancer mortality as the rest of the American population. Further research showed that when Japanese moved here, they quickly adapted our diet and abandoned their traditional soy foods.

Researchers have recently discovered that soybeans are a veritable pharmacy of anticancer chemicals, each with unique properties. For example, one compound found in soybeans, genistein, can block the spread of cancerous tumors by preventing the growth of new blood vessels to nourish the cancer cells. Test tube studies show that genistein is particularly effective in thwarting the growth of prostate and breast cancer cells. In fact, genistein is now being used as an experimental treatment for both types of cancers. Soy also contains isoflavones—weak, estrogenlike compounds that modulate the effects of the stronger estrogen and testosterone produced by the body. There is no evidence that estrogen and testosterone cause cancer, but they can trigger the growth of existing breast and prostate tumors. Daidzein, an isoflavone in soy, may be especially beneficial to women in controlling the effects of potent estrogens that could stimulate the growth of breast cancer cells. Soy is also rich in phytic acid, a potent antioxidant, as well as protease inhibitors, compounds that inhibit the action of tumor-promoting enzymes. With every bite of soy, you are getting an arsenal against cancer.

There is yet another good reason to get more soy in your life: it can protect against heart disease. According to an analysis of 38 medical studies undertaken by James W. Anderson, M.D., of the University of Kentucky, the daily consumption of 47 grams of soy protein can significantly lower total cholesterol levels and reduce high blood triglycerides. Although I have spent a great deal of time talking about cancer, it is important to remember that heart disease is still the number one killer in the United States and should be of concern to everyone.

Recently, women in midlife have discovered that the plant estrogens in soy can help relieve the symptoms of menopause, such as hot flashes, irritability, and vaginal dryness. In one Australian study, 58 postmenopausal women who had at least 14 hot flashes a week were given 45 grams of soy flour daily in the form of baked goods. Within a six-week period, women taking soy flour reported a 40 percent decline in hot flashes.

Despite all the good publicity about soy foods, few Americans eat enough of them. I love soy foods and eat a few ounces of tofu or drink a soy milk shake every day, but I understand that to many Americans, soy is simply not palatable. The good news is that you can now get all the benefits of soy by simply swallowing a pill or drinking a powdered beverage. A new generation of standardized soy concentrate supplements containing genistein, daidzein, isoflavones and other important cancer fighting agents are now in natural food stores. Sprouted soy concentrate is a particularly potent source of these important phyto-estrogens.

POSSIBLE BENEFITS

May prevent breast, prostate, and possibly other cancers.
Lowers elevated cholesterol and triglycerides.
May relieve symptoms of menopause.

THE RIGHT AMOUNT

Drink one soy protein shake daily. Make sure it contains genistein and daidzein.
Take two tablets daily. Be sure the soy concentrate supplement contains genistein and daidzein. (The usual dose is 10 mg. of genistein and daidzein, along with other isoflavones.)

Personal Advice

I take a combination of soy isoflavones (daidzein and genistein), plus calcium, magnesium, vitamin D, and boron to prevent osteoporosis. This blend is also excellent for relieving menopausal symptoms.

Suma

FACTS

Known as "para todo," meaning "for everything," suma is the dried root of the *Pfaffia paniculata* plant, native to the rainforest of Brazil. Even though suma has been used for more than a decade in the United States, it is just now gaining in popularity and is being included in many combination formulas designed to increase energy, stamina, and immune function. Suma is not necessarily taken for a specific medical problem; rather, it is used to improve overall health and vitality. Like other tonic herbs such as ginseng, suma is reputed to be an adaptogen—that is, an herb that helps enhance the body's reaction to stress, improves resistance against infection, and keeps the body running in peak condition. Japanese researchers performed comparative studies with suma and ginseng and found that the two herbs were so similar in structure and function that they dubbed suma "Brazilian ginseng."

Suma contains several biologically active compounds that have proven value for health, including allantoin, which promotes growth by stimulating protein synthesis and boosts immune function. Because of its anabolic action (it stimulates growth), suma is used to accelerate the healing of bone fractures and wounds. Suma also contains high levels of germanium (another Hot 100 supplement), vitamins, minerals, and hormone-like compounds. Body builders and athletes use suma to improve their workouts and speed recovery from injury.

In Brazil, suma is considered serious medicine. It has cancer-fighting substances called pfaffosides, which can inhibit the growth of melanoma cells in culture, and it has been used as a treatment for various types of cancer. Natural healers prescribe suma to patients with chronic fatigue syndrome and other problems typical of poor immune function.

Suma's reputation has spread by word of mouth; there are few scientific studies to back up these claims. However, this herb has been used for centuries by rainforest inhabitants, and it is an important part of their traditional healing practices.

POSSIBLE BENEFITS

Helps keep body functioning in peak condition.
May speed up recovery from wounds and fractures.
May be an anticarcinogen.
Strengthens immune function.

THE RIGHT AMOUNT

Take up to three 500-mg. capsules daily.

Taurine

FACTS

Taurine is a nonessential amino acid, which means that the body can synthesize it on its own. Taurine is abundant in the tissues of the heart, the skeletal muscles, and the central nervous system. It is essential for the proper digestion of fats, the absorption of fat-soluble vitamins, and the production of bile salts. Recently, researchers have found exciting new uses for taurine that have earned it a place on the Hot 100.

One particularly intriguing use for taurine is for heart failure, a serious condition that is often very difficult to treat. Heart failure means that the heart muscle can't effectively pump blood throughout the body. When the heart muscle becomes sluggish, the blood backs up, and this can lead to swelling in the legs and fluid retention in the lungs. Like prescription drugs such as digitalis, taurine can enhance the contractile action of the heart, which makes the heart pump more forcefully. In Japan, where natural remedies such as coenzyme-Q10 (see page 32) are often used for heart disease, physicians use taurine to treat heart failure. In fact, in one 1992 study involving 17 patients with heart failure, physicians reported that patients given taurine for heart failure showed greater improvement than those given coenzyme-Q10. In the United States, innovative alternative physicians are already recommending taurine to patients with heart disease to prevent heart failure. If you have a heart condition, do not try to self-medicate; work with a knowledgeable physician or natural healer.

Taurine is not just good for your heart; there is intriguing new evidence that it may also be good for your eyes. Animal studies have shown that when fed a taurine-deficient diet, animals will develop macular degeneration, destruction of the macula, the part of the retina that is responsible for central vision. In humans, macular degeneration is the leading cause of blindness in people over 50. Taurine may prevent macular degeneration by protecting the rods and cones, specialized cells in the retina that are instrumental in vision. This is especially important for diabetics, who are particularly vulnerable to macular degeneration. Although the cause of macular degeneration is unknown, it is probably related to oxidative damage and free radical damage from exposure to ultraviolet rays. Taurine, along with antioxidants, zinc, and herbs such as bilberry, is often included in special formulas designed to bolster vision.

POSSIBLE BENEFITS

Strengthens heart function.
May prevent macular degeneration.

THE RIGHT AMOUNT

Take up to three 500-mg. capsules daily.

Trimethylglycine (TMG)

FACTS

Trimethylglycine (TMG), also known as betaine, is a naturally occurring substance found in plants and animals, especially in beets, broccoli, and spinach. TMG is a wonderful source of methyl groups, molecules consisting of one carbon atom and three hydrogen atoms. In a process called methylation, methyl groups deactivate harmful substances in the body, converting them into helpful substances.

Homocysteine, an amino acid in the body, is one of the potentially harmful substances that is controlled by methyl groups. By now, you probably know that high levels of homocysteine can increase the risk of heart disease. According to the Physician's Health Study, conducted by researchers at Harvard, men with high homocysteine levels have three times more risk of having a heart attack than those with lower levels. Other studies have linked high homocysteine levels to an increased risk of birth defects, depression, certain forms of cancer, and even Alzheimer's disease. Clearly, high homocysteine levels are a threat to your health. Fortunately, it is relatively easy to lower your homocysteine levels by taking methyl-rich TMG. The methyl groups in TMG can convert harmful homocysteine into methionine, a beneficial amino acid.

Eating a diet rich in fruits and vegetables, and steering clear of processed foods, can also help reduce homocysteine levels. On the other hand, smoking, eating high amounts of saturated fat, and taking birth control pills will increase them.

As we age, methylation in the body declines, which means that homocysteine levels are allowed to rise. Not so coincidentally, there is also an increased risk of developing heart disease, cancer, and other health problems associated with elevated homocysteine levels. In earlier books, I have also recommended taking folic acid, a B vitamin, to help reduce the level of homocysteine. Folic acid is another wonderful source of methyl groups, as is vitamin B_{12}.

POSSIBLE BENEFITS

Reduces risk of heart disease.
Prevents certain forms of cancer.
Protects against Alzheimer's disease and depression.

THE RIGHT AMOUNT

Take three 100-mg. tablets daily.

Personal Advice

Omega-3 fatty acids, found in fish and flaxseed oil, have also been shown to reduce the levels of homocysteine.

Vanadyl Sulfate

FACTS

Vanadyl sulfate is a biologically active form of vanadium, a trace mineral that mimics the action of the hormone insulin. Produced by specialized cells in the pancreas, insulin regulates the metabolism of carbohydrate and protein, breaking down these nutrients into a form that can be utilized by the cells to make energy. If you don't produce enough insulin, or develop a condition called insulin resistance (in which the cells become resistant to insulin), your body will be unable to maintain normal blood sugar levels.

Because of its insulin-like properties, vanadyl is being used by progressive alternative physicians and natural healers to treat diabetes, characterized by excess sugar in the blood and urine. Studies show that vanadyl is very effective in normalizing blood sugar levels and controlling conditions such as insulin resistance, or Type II diabetes, which is becoming widespread in the United States and is associated with an increased risk of obesity, heart disease, gallbladder disease, and other medical conditions. (People with Type II diabetes produce enough insulin, but it works less efficiently.) If you have diabetes or elevated blood sugar, however, do not self-medicate with vanadyl or any other supplement. In some cases, vanadyl can lower blood sugar levels too quickly, causing serious problems. Your best bet is to work with a knowledgeable physician.

Recently, vanadyl sulfate has become one of the most popular supplements among athletes and body builders on the assumption that any substance that helps improve nutrient transport into the cells will increase the production of energy throughout the body and stimulate the growth of muscle tissue. Serious body builders swear that within two or three weeks of taking vanadyl sulfate, they feel and see a real difference in the size and strength of their muscles. To date, there have not been any serious studies to support this claim, but I've heard these anecdotes from enough people to believe that it warrants serious consideration. If vanadyl sulfate works as well to build muscle as body builders claim, it might also be useful for the very sick or for elderly people who suffer from muscle loss. Certainly, more studies need to be done on this interesting mineral.

POSSIBLE BENEFITS

Can help to control blood sugar levels in diabetics.
May help build muscle, increasing strength and definition.

THE RIGHT AMOUNT

If you have diabetes and want to try vanadyl sulfate, you must follow your doctor's instructions. He or she should monitor you closely until your blood sugar levels are normalized.
For body building, the usual dose is 10 mg. half an hour before working out.

CAUTIONS

High levels of trace minerals can be toxic. Do not exceed the recommended doses.

Personal Advice

There are so many new and interesting sports supplements on the market that there is absolutely no reason for any athlete to risk the potential hazards of steroids! Steroids dampen your immune system, weaken your bones, change your personality, and can cause severe medical and psychological problems. Not all sports supplements will work for everybody, but if you persevere, you will find the ones that are right for you.

Whey

FACTS

Can taking the right protein supplement enhance and extend your life? There's compelling evidence that it can. Protein is essential for normal growth, cell repair, and the production of hormones, immune cells, and muscle. Recently, scientists have begun to investigate the health benefits of a particular type of protein: whey protein concentrate, which is derived from milk protein. Unlike whole milk, whey protein concentrate does not contain fat, lactose (a milk sugar that can be hard to digest), or any other undesirable ingredients. What it does contain, however, are six different types of protein that have potent disease-fighting properties.

Numerous studies have shown that whey protein can enhance immune function in animals and is highly effective against common infections such as *Salmonella* infection and *Streptococcus* pneumonia. More importantly, whey protein concentrate can raise blood levels of glutathione, the body's primary antioxidant, which is found in virtually every cell. Glutathione not only protects us against free radical attack but is instrumental in a well-functioning immune system. As we age, our levels of glutathione decline, which many researchers believe may be why we are more vulnerable to disease. For example, people with Alzheimer's disease have lower levels of glutathione than people who do not, a finding that has led many researchers to surmise that glutathione must play a protective role against this degenerative disease. Glutathione supplements are not easily absorbed by the body; therefore, any substance that can boost glutathione is of great value.

Whether through its glutathione-enhancing effect or some other mechanism, concentrated whey protein can significantly extend life, at least in laboratory animals. According to studies performed at the University of Nebraska Medical Center, hamsters fed whey protein lived 60 percent longer than hamsters fed the usual animal chow. If concentrated whey protein works only half as well on humans, we can all look forward to living well past 100!

When you are shopping at your local natural food store, you may have noticed several brands of concentrated whey protein in the sports supplement section. Body builders and athletes place such high demands on their bodies that they need additional protein to help maintain existing muscle and build new muscle. However, given all the potential benefits of concentrated whey protein, I can wholeheartedly recommend it for couch potatoes.

POSSIBLE BENEFITS

Raises blood levels of glutathione.
Improves immune function.
May extend life.

THE RIGHT AMOUNT

Dissolve 2 tablespoons (1 ounce) in ½ cup of water or juice daily.

Yohimbe

FACTS

This herb is so hot that retailers tell me it is practically walking off the shelves at natural food stores. No wonder: It is being touted as the herb that can make men sexier and stronger. It is reputed to boost male potency as well as build muscle—a promise few men can resist. It's important to know, however, that a great deal of hype surrounds yohimbe, and before you use it you need to know the facts.

Yohimbe, extracted from the bark of a tree native to West Africa, has long been a folk remedy for impotence and used as an aphrodisiac by natural healers. A stronger version of yohimbe, yohimbine hydrochloride, is an FDA-approved treatment for impotence, the inability to have or maintain an erection, and is available by prescription only. Yohimbine hydrochloride dilates the blood vessels, thereby improving the flow of blood to the penis. Studies show that for at least half the men who use it, yohimbine can be useful in increasing potency. The problem is that yohimbine hydrochloride can cause a sudden drop in blood pressure, which can be dangerous, and it should not be used at all by people who have low blood pressure or heart problems, or who are taking antidepressant medication. In some cases, yohimbine hydrochloride can even cause anxiety attacks, which is certainly not conducive to good sex.

The weaker yohimbe herbal products can be purchased over the counter. There are no scientific studies to back up the claim that these products can improve sexual function; however, there are anecdotal reports from men who claim that they can work wonders. Many combination products designed to improve sexual performance for men include yohimbe, along with ginkgo biloba, zinc, and L-arginine. Since yohimbine hydrochloride can cause serious side effects in some men, I err on the side of caution with yohimbe. Before you use it, I recommend that you check with your physician or natural healer.

What about the claims that yohimbe can help body builders bulk up? They are based on the mistaken notion that since yohimbe can enhance sexual function, it must do so by increasing the level of testosterone, the primary male hormone, which not only is involved in sexual response but can also stimulate the growth of muscle. There is no evidence, however, that yohimbe has any effect on hormone levels or on muscle building. If you are looking to increase your strength and stamina, there are better sports supplements that can help you accomplish those goals.

POSSIBLE BENEFITS

May enhance libido and improve sexual performance.

THE RIGHT AMOUNT

Take one to three 500-mg. capsules daily. Talk to your physician or natural healer to find the dose that is right for you.

CAUTION

Use this herb under the guidance of a medical professional.

Personal Advice

Most cases of impotence in men are caused by atherosclerosis, or hardening of the arteries, which impairs the blood flow to the penis. Paying attention to your cardiovascular health, maintaining normal levels of blood lipids, eating enough fruits and vegetables, and taking antioxidant supplements to prevent lipid problems is the best way to stay healthy, strong, and sexy!

Zeaxanthin

FACTS

I launched the Hot 100 with alpha carotene, one of 500 carotenoids that provide natural color in plants and do so much more. I end with zeaxanthin, another antioxidant carotenoid that is making headlines because it may help prevent a leading cause of blindness among older people: macular degeneration.

The macula is a tiny dimple on the retina that is responsible for fine vision. Damage to the macula can cause blurry vision, or a dark spot in the field of vision. It can eventually lead to a loss of central vision, which can make it impossible to read, drive, or operate a computer. There is no cure for macular degeneration, but in some cases surgery may help to slow its progress. Free radical damage from ultraviolet radiation is believed to be a contributing factor, if not the cause, of macular degeneration. In fact, studies have shown lower than normal blood levels of protective antioxidants in people who develop macular degeneration.

The good news is that some carotenoids appear to protect against this disease. According to a 1994 study conducted by five eye centers in the United States, people who ate foods with the highest amounts of two carotenoids—zeaxanthin and lutein (see page 97)—had the lowest risk of developing macular degeneration. Zeaxanthin may help protect the macula by blocking the activity of peroxide free radicals, guarding cell membranes against free radical damage. The problem, though, is that zeaxanthin is found in high concentration in watercress, Swiss chard, chicory leaf, beet greens, and okra—vegetables that are not particularly popular in this country. If you don't regularly eat these foods, you should consider taking a carotenoid supplement with zeaxanthin, or one of the new combination formulas designed to enhance vision that includes zeaxanthin.

Because of its antioxidant properties, zeaxanthin may also protect against various forms of cancer that can be initiated by free radical activity. In fact, preliminary studies show that zeaxanthin can decrease the rate of growth of tumor cells.

POSSIBLE BENEFITS

Helps protects against macular degeneration.
May help prevent cancer.

THE RIGHT AMOUNT

Take 30 to 130 mg. daily in a mixed carotenoid or antioxidant formula.

2

Hot News About Old Favorites

STOPS THE GROWTH OF PROSTATE CANCER CELLS

Used for more than 4,000 years as an herbal medicine, garlic may prove to be the wonder drug of the next millennium. Garlic is a "broad-spectrum" herb that offers numerous benefits. It is a natural antibiotic—in fact, during World War II when penicillin was scarce, the Russian army relied on garlic to prevent infection on the battlefield. Garlic can protect against heart disease by thwarting the formation of blood clots.

But there's even more exciting news about the herb known as the "stinking rose." According to researchers at New York's Memorial Sloan-Kettering Cancer Research Center, aged garlic can dramatically reduce the growth of human prostate cancer cells in test tube experiments. Researchers exposed prostate cancer cells to S-allylmercaptocysteine, a sulfur compound found only in aged (not fresh) garlic. Prostate cancer cells are sensitive to the male hormone testosterone and particularly to DHT, a potent metabolite of testosterone that can stimulate the growth of prostate tumors. When exposed to aged garlic, the cancer cells broke down testosterone two to four times faster than normal, and even better, did so through a pathway that does not produce the troublesome DHT.

In addition, the aged garlic reduced the body's production of prostate-specific antigen (PSA) which can cause prostate cells to grow. Higher than normal levels of PSA (over 4) may be a marker for prostate cancer or other problems. Prostate cancer is very common among older men, and there are few effective treatments. In fact, the treatment of choice is often no treatment, or a period of "watchful waiting" during which the patient is closely monitored by his physician. If the cancer stays contained, the patient may never need treatment. However, during this period of watchful waiting, I think it makes enormous sense to make positive changes in your lifestyle. Eliminating fatty foods, eating fresh vegetables, and adding soy foods to your diet are wonderful ways to improve your health and perhaps even prevent prostate cancer from progressing beyond its earliest stages. Adding garlic capsules to your diet also makes good sense. In fact, I urge all men to make these positive changes *before* they are confronted with prostate cancer. Researchers caution that fresh garlic won't do; the bulbs must be aged for at least a year. Aged garlic pills and capsules sold over the counter are a good source of this all-important cancer-fighting sulfur compound.

THE RIGHT AMOUNT

Take one raw, aged, odorless garlic capsule daily.

Capsaicin Cream

A CURE FOR YOUR PAIN IN THE NECK!

Capsaicin cream, to be used *only* externally, is derived from the active ingredient in hot chili peppers that gives them their characteristic bite. Marketed under several different names, capsaicin cream is fast becoming a favorite over-the-counter remedy for joint pain associated with arthritis. Researchers at Walter Reed Army Medical Center in Washington, D.C., now report that it is also a useful treatment for chronic neck pain. In their study, patients with chronic neck pain used a 0.025 percent capsaicin cream on the painful area four times daily. After five weeks, most patients reported significant improvement, and some were virtually free of pain.

How does capsaicin work? When applied to the skin, capsaicin cream creates a hot, burning sensation that stimulates nerve cells to release a chemical called substance P, which in turn triggers pain impulses. Once the nerve cells are depleted of substance P, the pain is diminished. It may take several days to a week, however, before you experience a noticeable reduction in pain. Although most people are able to tolerate the temporary discomfort caused by capsaicin cream, some may find it to be too irritating. If the pain of the capsaicin cream is intolerable, discontinue use.

THE RIGHT AMOUNT

To use capsaicin cream for arthritis or neck pain, massage the cream into the affected areas four times daily. Start with the lowest dose cream (0.025 percent), and if that is not effective within a week, try a higher dose (0.075 percent).

Reishi Mushroom

TRY THE VERSATILE "MEDICINE OF KINGS" FOR PAIN RELIEF

Known in China as the medicine of kings, and studied extensively by the Japanese, reishi mushroom has been highly prized for over 2,000 years by Asian healers, especially for its positive effect on heart function. Dubbed the elixir of life by Chinese healers, reishi has been prescribed for hundreds of years for people suffering from angina, or chest pain. This traditional use has been vindicated by current studies that show reishi to indeed be a potent cardiotonic. This special mushroom can improve blood flow to the heart, lower cholesterol, reduce high blood pressure, and prevent the formation of blood clots. For the past decade, reishi has also been used as a cancer treatment in Japan, with some success. Reishi appears to inhibit cancer via its beneficial effect on the immune system. Compounds in reishi can boost immune function by activating macrophages and T-cells, the disease-fighting cells that help rid the body of all foreign invaders, including viruses, bacteria, and cancer cells.

Recently, studies have revealed that reishi is also an analgesic: it can relieve pain for a wide variety of conditions and also reduce the anxiety that is often associated with chronic pain. Researchers at the University of Texas Health Science Center in San Antonio report that reishi is a natural anti-inflammatory agent that is effective in treating stiff necks, shoulder aches, and other joint problems. Reishi is also a time-honored remedy for insomnia, which makes a great deal of sense, since discomfort or pain makes it difficult to sleep well. For all of these reasons, I believe that reishi may prove to be an important treatment for arthritis and related conditions along with other natural treatments, such as sea cucumber, glucosamine sulfate, chondroitin sulfates, and essential fatty acids.

Reishi is available as tea and in capsules.

THE RIGHT AMOUNT

To relieve pain and inflammation, take 100 mg. extract of reishi daily.

If you have cancer, you should work with a knowledgeable physician or natural healer. As a cancer treatment, doses are much higher than those for pain control—you will need to take about 10 grams of reishi daily. But reishi is considered safe even at the highest levels; there is no known toxicity.

Vitamin D

SAVE YOUR KNEES WITH VITAMIN D

Can vitamins protect against osteoarthritis? According to a study performed at Tufts University Medical School, the answer is yes, especially if the vitamin in question is vitamin D. As part of the Framingham Heart Study, 500 men and women had knee x-rays to check for arthritis in the 1980s, and again eight years later. Diet and vitamin D blood levels were also tracked. In a study published in *Arthritis and Rheumatism* in 1996, researchers reported that people who had the highest levels of vitamin D intake had the smallest amount of disease progression over the eight-year period. Conversely, those with the lowest intake of vitamin D were the most likely to develop serious osteoarthritis in their knee joints.

Vitamin D is known as the "sunshine vitamin" because ultraviolet (UV) rays from the sun stimulate skin oils to produce vitamin D. Vitamin D is also found in foods such as fortified dairy products and fatty fish oils. Many people are deficient in vitamin D, especially those who live in northern climates that may not get adequate sunshine. (Remember, all you need is just a few minutes in the sun each day to produce vitamin D. I am not advocating sunbathing, which can cause skin cancer.)

THE RIGHT AMOUNT

Take one 400-IU of vitamin D daily. Do not exceed recommended dose.

Gamma Linolenic Acid (GLA)

AN OLD "NEW" TREATMENT FOR ARTHRITIS

For years, I've been recommending gamma linolenic acid (GLA), a fatty acid found in borage oil, as a treatment for arthritis. (Linolenic acid is similar to linoleic acid, another essential fatty acid critical for good health.) Finally, a study performed at the University of Massachusetts Medical Center confirms that GLA can reduce the aches and pains of arthritis, but without the side effects normally associated with other pain medications. In the year-long study, reported in the November 1996 issue of *Arthritis and Rheumatism*, 56 men and women took either GLA capsules (2.4 grams daily) or a placebo along with their regular prescription arthritis drugs for six months. Those taking the GLA were six times more likely to have significant improvement in joint pain and swelling than those taking the placebo; in the latter subjects, symptoms remained the same or even worsened. For the second six months, all patients were given GLA capsules. At the end of the year, half of the people using GLA experienced a 50 percent reduction in symptoms such as pain and stiffness. In fact, about 12 percent of the participants were able to reduce their dosage of prescription drugs after using GLA. GLA did not work overnight—it took several weeks before people experienced any real pain relief—but for most of the participants, their patience paid off.

THE RIGHT AMOUNT

The doses used in this study were exceedingly high. I believe that a good result can be achieved by taking a smaller dose, particularly if you are using other natural remedies. Take up to three 250-mg. capsules daily.

Ginseng

FACTS

You've seen it advertised on television as a new and exciting supplement that can rejuvenate and reinvigorate like none other. In reality, ginseng, an ancient herb grown in North America and Asia, is as old as recorded history. Ginseng first became popular in the West in the 1970s, when it was reported that Russian athletes used it to maintain their competitive edge. Russian scientists claimed that ginseng could improve strength, stamina, and concentration—all attributes required for competitive sports. The fact that Russian athletes performed so well in international competitions—and often far outperformed Western athletes—reinforced ginseng's reputation. Interest in ginseng began to wane as newer and more high-tech sports supplements were brought to market. Today, however, ginseng is enjoying a revival and is being marketed to baby boomers as an antidote to aging.

Ginseng is a tonic herb designed to enhance health and well-being. In herbal language, ginseng is an adaptogen—a word used to describe supplements that help the body perform at optimal levels and counter the ill effects of stress. Numerous studies have shown that ginseng can increase energy and alertness, strengthen immune function, and help relieve stress. It can also inhibit the growth of cancerous tumors in animals. A rich source of phytoestrogen, ginseng is used by many women to counteract the symptoms of menopause, such as hot flashes. There are several different types of ginseng: Panax ginseng is from Korea, American ginseng is grown here, and Siberian ginseng is actually a botanical cousin of Panax ginseng. The biologically active ingredients in American and Asian ginseng are ginsenosides. In Siberian ginseng, the biologically active ingredients are called eleutherosides.

Because many suppliers and manufacturers are unscrupulous, as much as 10 percent of all products that purport to be ginseng are nothing more than poor imitations. Your best bet is to purchase your ginseng from companies that you trust. If you use Asian or American ginseng, look for products containing 4 to 7 percent ginsenosides; for Siberian ginseng, look for products that contain eleutherosides equal to 1 percent of the total weight.

THE RIGHT AMOUNT

Take up to six 500-mg. capsules daily.

CAUTION

Avoid products combining ginseng with another herbal stimulant, ma huang (ephedra); these products make some people jittery. Ditto for caffeine: if you take ginseng, restrict your intake of caffeinated beverages.

German studies suggest that Siberian ginseng may aggravate severe high blood pressure and therefore should not be used by people with this condition. People with insomnia should steer clear of American and Asian ginseng because it may be too stimulating. Siberian ginseng, however, has a more gentle effect and is often used as a treatment for insomnia.

Personal Advice

Anyone who is interested in herbal medicine should know about the wonderful work performed by the American Botanical Council. Its magazine, *HerbalGram*, is an excellent source of information on the latest scientific research on herbs from around the world. (To contact the American Botanical Council, call 512-331-8868.)

Omega-3 Fatty Acids

REDUCE YOUR RISK OF BREAST CANCER

There is some compelling new evidence that omega-3 fatty acids may help prevent breast cancer and may even be a useful treatment for this disease. Several studies have already documented that omega-3 fatty acids from fatty fish (like salmon, sea bass, and mackerel) or from flaxseed oil can inhibit the growth of breast cancer cells in test tubes. It is also well known that Asian women, who are much less likely to get breast cancer than Western women, eat vast amounts of omega-3 fatty acids in their diet. Interestingly, Asian women also have a high concentration of omega-3 fatty acids in their breast tissue, while American women—who typically eat polyunsaturated vegetable oils consisting primarily of omega-6 fatty acids—have higher amounts of omega-6 oils in their breast tissue. This may be problematic, because animal studies suggest that the kind of polyunsaturated oils that are eaten in the West may actually increase the risk of breast cancer. In fact, studies have shown that women with breast cancer have a two- to five-fold higher ratio of omega-6 to omega-3.

These facts recently led researchers to explore whether omega-3 fatty acids could be an effective treatment for breast cancer. In one study conducted at the Johnson Cancer Center at the University of California, 25 women who had already been diagnosed with breast cancer volunteered to consume a diet that mirrored the Asian diet. Instead of eating the typical American "meat and potatoes" fare, for three months these women ate soy foods and leafy green vegetables, and they took fish oil supplements daily. At the end of the study, researchers detected a change in the composition of the breast tissue of the women on the diet. They had higher levels of omega-3 fatty acids and lower levels of omega-6 fatty acids than before they began the special diet. Researchers hope that these changes will protect these women from having a recurrence, and larger studies are currently under way.

Although it may be years before the scientific community agrees that omega-3 fatty acids may play a role in preventing breast cancer, as far as I'm concerned, given the high rate of breast cancer in the United States, it makes sense for you to do all you can to protect yourself. Adding fish oil supplements to your diet is easy enough to do, and there is virtually no downside. (Don't overdose on fish oil, however—too much can interfere with normal blood clotting. Stick to my recommended doses.) It also goes without saying that eating fish instead of meat is another good lifestyle choice.

THE RIGHT AMOUNT

Take up to six 1000-mg. capsules daily.

CAUTION

If you are taking blood thinners, such as coumadin or heparin, do not use omega-3 fatty acids unless advised by your physician.

Vitamin E

SLOWS DOWN ALZHEIMER'S DISEASE— STRENGTHENS IMMUNITY

Vitamin E was discovered more than 50 years ago, yet it seems we learn something new about this extraordinary antioxidant practically every day. Numerous studies have already proved that people who take vitamin E supplements are much less likely to get heart disease than those who don't. In one famous study reported in the *New England Journal of Medicine* in May 1993, researchers monitored 87,000 registered female nurses and 40,000 male health professionals for eight years. In both studies, those who consumed at least 100 IU of vitamin E supplements daily had a 40 percent reduced risk of heart disease. In fact, many cardiologists are now routinely prescribing this vitamin for their patients.

Now, there is even more good news about vitamin E, this time in connection with Alzheimer's disease. Recently, the *New England Journal of Medicine* reported on a study in which 341 patients with early Alzheimer's disease of moderate severity were given either a prescription drug, vitamin E (2000 IU), a combination of both, or a placebo for two years. The purpose of the study was to determine whether any of the treatments could slow down the progress of the disease, which in its most severe form can cause severe mental deterioration and the inability to perform even the simplest of tasks. After evaluating the patients at the end of the study, the researchers concluded that the risk of reaching the primary endpoint—the most severe stage of Alzheimer's disease—was 53 percent lower in the vitamin E group, 43 percent lower in the drug group, and 31 percent lower in the group receiving combination therapy than the placebo group. Clearly, the results were overwhelmingly in favor of vitamin E.

Vitamin E can also help to prevent the decline in immune function that typically occurs in older people. As we age, our immune systems age too. Our immune cells don't work as efficiently as when we are young, and as a result, we are more vulnerable to infection. A cold that we could once shake off in a day or two can linger for weeks. The flu, which can be nothing more than a nuisance in a young person, can quickly turn deadly in an older person. One sign of a weakened immune function in older people is that vaccinations often don't "take" as well as they do in the young. A vaccination is a weakened form of a virus that is introduced into the body so that the immune system can respond by producing antibodies against it. If the vaccination is effective, an army of antibodies is ready to pounce on the virus if it encounters it again. However, because of their sluggish immune systems, older people do not always respond strongly to vaccinations. Recently, Dr. Simin Meydani, a well-known vitamin E researcher at Tufts University, gave either vitamin E supplements ranging from 60 to 800 IU or a placebo to 88 healthy people aged 65 or older daily for four months. Those who took 200 IU of vitamin E or more daily showed a significant improvement in immune function, as demonstrated by a stronger response to the hepatitis B vaccine than those who had been taking the placebo. In fact, those who took the vitamin E produced six times more antibodies to the hepatitis B vaccine than those taking the placebo. In addition, everyone taking vitamin E showed improvement in immune function in other areas. The message is an obvious one: take your vitamin E!

THE RIGHT AMOUNT

Take 400 IU of vitamin E daily. If you are over 40, use the dry form (succinate) of vitamin E because it is better absorbed.

Ginkgo Biloba

IMPROVES CIRCULATION FOR BETTER SEX, BETTER MEMORY

Dating back to the Ice Age, the ginkgo biloba tree is well known for its longevity: it is not uncommon for a tree to live to be 1,000! Although it is relatively new in the United States, ginkgo biloba is the most widely prescribed medication in Europe, often for problems related to poor circulation. Every system of the body—from the brain to sexual function—is dependent on a steady supply of blood, which provides both oxygen and nutrients to hungry cells. If the blood flow is compromised, we will feel the effects in countless ways, leaving us feeling both physically and mentally fatigued.

Ginkgo can help reverse these problems by restoring adequate circulation. For example, in a study reported in the *British Journal of Clinical Pharmacology* in 1992, researchers noted that 120 to 160 mg. per day of ginkgo biloba extract could enhance circulation to the brain, which in turn helped to improve memory and concentration in volunteers. Ginkgo biloba has also been used successfully to treat male sexual problems caused by inadequate blood flow to the penis, a major cause of erectile dysfunction. In one study reported in *Urology*, 50 impotent men were given 240 mg. of ginkgo biloba for nine months. In addition, some of the men were also given papaverine, a muscle stimulant that can improve erections. Researchers reported that the ginkgo biloba supplement greatly improved erections in both groups, whether or not the men had also taken papaverine.

Until recently, no one knew precisely how ginkgo affected circulation, but according to Dr. Lester Packer, a professor in the Department of Molecular and Cell Biology at the University of California at Berkeley, ginkgo's primary role in the body may be as a regulator of nitric oxide metabolism. Nitric oxide is critical for regulating many body functions, including blood flow. Although nitric oxide is essential, too much can be dangerous, and it has been linked to atherosclerosis (the hardening of the arteries) and other diseases. On the basis of Dr. Packer's research, ginkgo appears to help maintain nitric oxide at safe levels. Anyone with a circulatory problem—or who wants to avoid one—should take ginkgo biloba.

A study reported in *Radiology and Oncology* suggests that ginkgo biloba may also be a useful therapy for cancer. In the study, ginkgo biloba was administered to laboratory mice undergoing radiation therapy for fibrosarcoma of the leg muscle. The mice given ginkgo needed only 50 percent of the radiation to shrink their tumors as they would if they had not been given ginkgo biloba. The less radiation needed to do the job, the less likelihood of producing radiation burns, a common problem with radiation therapy. More studies are required to determine whether ginkgo biloba will work as well on humans undergoing radiation, but these early reports are extremely promising.

THE RIGHT AMOUNT

Take up to three 60-mg. capsules or tablets of standardized ginkgo biloba daily.

Licorice

NATURE'S ANTI-INFLAMMATORY AGENT

The Hot 100 includes a derivative of licorice called DGL, which is excellent for gastrointestinal disorders such as chronic indigestion and stomach ulcers (see page 45). DGL is a form of licorice that is stripped of glycyrrhetinic acid, a natural anti-inflammatory compound that under certain conditions can raise blood pressure. Therefore, if you have high blood pressure, I recommend that you do not use real licorice products but stick to DGL. But if blood pressure isn't a problem, licorice products may be beneficial.

For centuries, Asian healers have relied on licorice to treat arthritis, allergies, and other conditions that can be triggered by an inflammatory response. According to *HerbalGram*, a magazine that covers the latest medical news about herbs, Japanese researchers have reported that licorice may be an effective treatment for lupus, an autoimmune disease in which the body's immune cells attack its own tissue. Lupus is characterized by fatigue, arthritis-type joint pain, and a butterfly-type rash on the face, among other symptoms. In advanced cases, lupus can result in damage to vital organs. Unfortunately, there is no cure for lupus, and standard drug therapy often involves using corticosteroids (cortisone) or strong chemotherapy drugs to suppress immune function. Lupus patients typically have elevated levels of immune complexes, which indicate that the immune system is going into "overdrive." The good news is that researchers at the Oriental Medical Research Center in Tokyo found that licorice can normalize the levels of these potentially troublesome immune complexes in mice, which suggests that it may have a similar effect on humans.

Even though licorice helps control an overactive system, unlike corticosteroids it does not depress immune function, which can leave you vulnerable to infection. Licorice not only enhances immune function but does so safely, and it also has strong antiviral properties. Since numerous studies have shown that licorice can thwart the growth of cancerous tumors in animals, this herb is also being studied as a potential cancer treatment.

Recently I learned about another fascinating new use for this time-honored remedy. Israeli researchers have discovered that licorice contains a natural antioxidant that can help prevent atherosclerosis, or hardening of the arteries. The oxidation of LDL (or "bad" cholesterol) is believed to be a major cause of atherosclerosis, which can lead to a heart attack. In the study, 20 medical students were given 100-mg. tablets of licorice extract daily. Within two weeks, the LDL in their blood was more resistant to oxidation than people taking a placebo.

THE RIGHT AMOUNT

Take up to three 500-mg. capsules daily.

Magnesium

THE MIRACLE MINERAL FOR HEALTH AND ENERGY

Magnesium is a hard-working mineral that we take for granted. It's not hyped like many other supplements, nor is it considered to be on the cutting edge. Yet, the more we learn about magnesium, the more we realize that the effects of this mineral are nothing short of miraculous.

Magnesium is involved in nearly every essential bodily function, from the beating of the heart to the creation of bone and the regulation of blood sugar. It is so important that it is called the "gatekeeper of cellular activity," signifying its critical role in cellular processes. Magnesium is abundant in foods such as wheat bran, almonds, and tofu, but most Americans do not get enough magnesium from food.

Magnesium is of particular importance to women, who often suffer magnesium deficiencies. Postmenopausal women, who are especially likely to be low in magnesium, are more vulnerable to dangerous blood clots, which can lead to heart attacks and stroke. In addition to increasing the risk of heart disease in women, low levels of magnesium contribute to another major health problem: osteoporosis. Pregnant women who are deficient in magnesium are prone to develop toxemia, a form of high blood pressure that is potentially lethal for themselves and their babies, and to deliver prematurely. Magnesium deficiency may also be a factor in premenstrual syndrome (PMS).

Magnesium helps to burn fat and produce energy, which is critical for both men and women. If you are feeling tired and are getting flabby, it could be a sign of magnesium deficiency. A study conducted at the USDA's

Grand Forks Human Nutrition Research Center found that postmenopausal women with low magnesium levels had less energy and did not burn fat efficiently, making physical exertion more difficult. This can lead to a vicious circle: "I can't exercise because I'm so tired—but because I'm not exercising, I'm gaining weight and feeling even more tired." The solution? Make sure that you are getting enough magnesium.

Heavy drinkers often have low levels of magnesium, which may be why alcohol abuse is associated with an increased risk of heart disease and osteoporosis.

THE RIGHT AMOUNT

Take 250–500 mg. (tablets) daily. (For each 250 mg. of magnesium, take 500 mg. of calcium.)

Selenium

CANCER FIGHTER

Selenium, a mineral concentrated in soil, is an antioxidant that is critical for the production of glutathione peroxidase, the body's primary antioxidant that is found in every cell. An exciting new study sponsored by the National Cancer Institute suggests that selenium supplements can greatly reduce the risk of cancer. In the study, 1,312 patients with a history of skin cancer were given either 200 mcg. of selenium daily or a placebo and were monitored for eight years. Initially, the study was established to determine whether selenium would prevent a recurrence of skin cancer.

At first glance, the researchers were disappointed because selenium did not appear to protect against future skin cancers. Much to their astonishment, however, the selenium takers had significantly lower rates of other kinds of cancer, including those affecting the lung, prostate, and colon. In fact, the group taking the selenium had less than half the death rate from cancer as the group taking the placebo. (There were 29 cancer-related deaths among the selenium takers and 57 deaths among the placebo takers.) Researchers speculate that selenium's power over cancer may be purely preventive and that once cancer takes hold in the body, selenium may not be able to stop it from progressing.

This is not the first time that selenium has been linked to a lower rate of cancer and other diseases. Numerous studies have shown that people who have cancer, heart disease, or other serious illnesses have lower than normal levels of selenium and glutathione. Conversely, people with high blood levels of selenium are at a lower risk of developing cancer or having a stroke than people with low levels of this mineral. In fact, the southwestern United States is known as the "stroke belt" because it has the highest rate of stroke in the country and has the lowest levels of selenium in the soil.

Garlic, onions, broccoli, whole grains, and red grapes are excellent food sources of selenium, but Americans may not be getting enough of this mineral from food. As I noted earlier, the level of selenium in soil varies according to geographic area, and these disparities are reflected in the food grown from that soil. But even if food starts out selenium-rich, modern methods of food production can destroy this precious mineral. For example, processing wheat to white flour strips it of much of its selenium, a practice for which we may be paying a steep price. American men are five times more likely to die of prostate cancer than Japanese men; the difference in mortality rates could be because the Asian diet contains four times the amount of selenium as the average American diet. Of course, there are other foods in the Asian diet, such as soy, that may help reduce the risk of prostate cancer, but selenium also does appear to be a protective factor. Raising your blood level of selenium is not difficult: the more selenium you consume, the higher your blood levels. To me, taking selenium supplements, in addition to eating selenium-rich foods, is good insurance against disease.

POSSIBLE BENEFITS

Reduces risk of developing cancer, heart disease, or stroke.

THE RIGHT AMOUNT

Take between 100 and 200 mcg. daily.

3

Fat Burners and Sports Supplements

Two of the fastest-growing categories of new supplements are classified as either fat burners or sports supplements. Fat burners (sometimes called thermogenic stimulators or metabolic enhancers) are substances that speed up metabolism, thereby promoting the loss of fat. Sports supplements are substances that either build muscle, increase strength and stamina, or aid in recovery from exercise. In some cases, a sports supplement can also be a fat burner, and vice versa.

Although there are similarities between fat burners and sports supplements, there are also some important differences. Fat burners in general are for people who want to lose weight and maintain a sleek body. On the other hand, some—but not all—sports supplements are designed to help body builders "bulk up." In fact, these supplements are often high in calories and should be used only by people who engage in vigorous exercise with the specific goal of building muscle.

I don't want to leave you with the impression that sports supplements are only for body builders or competitive athletes who spend their days pumping iron. Not at all. In reality, many of these supplements are meant to be used by ordinary people who are enthusiastic about fitness and want to do all they can to improve their bodies. These folks typically may work out a few times a week, or enjoy sports on the weekends, but nevertheless are looking for an added boost.

In the not-too-distant past, sports supplements were a euphemism for anabolic steroids, hormone-like drugs that were available by prescription and could lead to serious health problems if abused, which they often were. The good news today is that the shelves of natural food stores are packed with nonsteroidal supplements that are not only quite effective but usually safe and all legal. I want to caution that some of the sports supplements that I write about, particularly those that boost testosterone levels, are new and untested. They *may* be perfectly safe, but we simply don't know their long-term effects. Use them with caution, especially if you have a family history of a hormone-dependent cancer, such as prostate cancer. (As a rule, women should be cautious about taking testosterone-boosting supplements. Although these supplements may build muscle, they can cause unwanted side effects such as facial hair. Testosterone may be given to postmenopausal women as part of hormone replacement therapy, but the dose is carefully controlled to reduce the risk of side effects.)

Do sports supplements and fat burners really work? No pill or potion will magically transform your body. All of these supplements are meant to work in synergy with exercise and a sensible eating regimen, but they cannot do the job alone.

The following is a review of some of the newest and hottest of these supplements.

Androstenedione

One of the most talked-about new sports supplements, androstenedione is primarily being used by male body builders and athletes. It is a metabolite of DHEA, a Hot 100 natural hormone produced by the body. Preliminary studies suggest that androstenedione may boost the body's level of testosterone, which may help build muscle.

Testosterone attracted the attention of body builders in 1996 when the *New England Journal of Medicine* reported on a study in which male weight lifters were given weekly testosterone injections or a placebo. Both groups of men engaged in the same exercise program. At the end of the ten weeks, the men taking testosterone had significantly bigger triceps and quadriceps than the men taking placebos. Testosterone, however, is available by prescription only and is not supposed to be used by men unless they are medically diagnosed with a testosterone deficiency. That is why body builders are looking to over-the-counter testosterone-boosting agents such as androstenedione to produce the same effect.

There is already much lore surrounding androstenedione, including stories that androstenedione had been widely used by East German athletes who performed so well in international competitions. There are few human studies to back up these claims, however, and some researchers are skeptical that androstenedione can really boost testosterone in a significant way. Many body builders contend, however, that it produces results.

Androstenedione is sold separately, but more often in combination with other sports supplements. Take two 100-mg. capsules daily; take one of those capsules one hour before working out.

Note: Testosterone is broken down into a more potent form called dihydrotestosterone, which can cause enlargement of the prostate and stimulate the growth of prostate tumors. If you have an enlarged prostate or prostate cancer, I would recommend not using this product, or any other that boosts testosterone levels. In addition, men using a testosterone-boosting agent should be sure to take saw palmetto (see page 154), an herb that protects prostate health.

Antioxidants for Recovery

Exercise does wonderful things for your body. It firms and tones your muscles, burns excess calories, and makes you feel energized from your head to your toes. There is, however, a price to pay for the benefits of exercise: The more you work out, the more oxygen you burn, and the more oxygen you burn, the more free radicals you are going to produce. Free radicals are what cause a charley horse, the sore, stiff feeling that often accompanies a rigorous workout a day or two later. Recent studies suggest that antioxidants can speed the recovery of muscles and reduce the post-workout blues.

Vitamins A, C, and E, as well as selenium, are well known antioxidants that I recommend taking whether or not you work out. Several new antioxidants, however, are gaining popularity among fitness mavens. Lipoic acid, which I discuss on page 94, is one of them. Not only is lipoic acid a potent antioxidant, it also helps to enhance energy production in the body and to normalize blood sugar levels. Take two 50-mg. capsules daily.

N-acetyl cysteine (NAC) (see page 114) is another supplement that can promote faster recovery after a workout. Studies show that supplemental NAC can replenish blood levels of glutathione, which in turn will reduce the level of free radicals in the blood and promote a quicker recovery. Take three 500-mg. capsules or tablets of NAC with meals.

Bromelain

An enzyme found in pineapple, bromelain can reduce pain and inflammation following injury and help muscles recover more quickly after a workout. Bromelain contains a natural anti-inflammatory agent and is also used to relieve pain caused by sprains and other athletic injuries. Take up to three 500-mg. tablets daily.

Chrysin

Although estrogen is known as a female hormone, and testosterone is known as a male hormone, in reality men produce a small amount of estrogen, and women produce a small amount of testosterone. In both men and women, testosterone is broken down into estrogen. In fact, one of the problems with men taking supplements to boost testostorone levels to build muscle is the possibility that the result will be higher levels of estrogen, which will have a feminizing effect. This is not exactly what the average body builder has in mind!

Chrysin, also known as flavone X, inhibits aromatase, an enzyme responsible for breaking down testosterone into estrogen, thereby helping to maintain higher testosterone levels. Chrysin can be taken alone or used along with other testosterone-boosting agents, such as androstenedione and DHEA. There are few human studies on chrysin; however, European Olympic athletes who took

1 to 3 grams of chrysin reportedly experienced a 30 percent increase in testosterone.

Caffeine, Ephedra and Other Stimulants

Caffeine is a thermogenic agent, meaning that it speeds up metabolism so that you burn calories faster. It is also a stimulant that increases energy (at least temporarily) and makes you more alert. Ephedra is an herb that has traditionally been used for respiratory problems and in fact is an ingredient in many antihistamines. Several weight-loss products combine caffeine with ephedra and possibly other thermogenic agents as well. My advice is to use these products with caution. Keep in mind that one cup of coffee contains up to 120 mg. of caffeine, and many of these diet formulas contain that much or more caffeine in just one capsule. Excess caffeine can cause insomnia, jitteriness, and heart palpitations. Ditto for ephedra, which can also raise blood pressure.

People respond differently to caffeine and ephedra. Some people may be highly sensitive to these stimulants, while others can use them with no adverse effects. Frankly, I'm not too keen on stimulants, but if you do use them, be careful not to overdo it. If you feel dizzy, anxious, or restless after using these products, discontinue use.

Avoid the thermogenic agents found in typical diet pills that contain amphetamine. These drugs not only can cause adverse reactions in many people but can be habit-forming.

Ciwuja

This Chinese herb is being touted as the sports supplement that can burn fat and enhance stamina. In different studies, researchers at the Academy of Preventive Medicine in Beijing, China, and the Department of Physiology at the University of North Texas Health Science Center discovered that ciwuja can alter normal metabolism during exercise so that you burn more fat and less carbohydrate. The promise is that if you take ciwuja, you can work out longer and harder before feeling tired. Ciwuja is sold separately or in combination sports formulas. (See page 31.)

Chromium Picolinate

Studies suggest that this mineral can help trim fat and build muscle, making this the supplement for body builders and regular folks who want to lose weight and firm up.

In one study conducted at Bemidji State University in Minnesota, male athletes took 200 mcg. daily or a placebo. After six weeks, the men taking chromium gained 44 percent more lean body mass, as opposed to only 7 percent in the placebo group.

In another study, sedentary overweight people who took chromium for 72 days lost an average of 4.2 fat pounds and gained 1.4 pounds in lean mass. What is particularly intriguing is that they achieved this result without cutting calories or exercising!

For these reasons, I recommend chromium to anyone who wants a sleeker, stronger body. Take between 200 and 600 mcg. of chromium picolinate daily.

Chitosan

"Fat blockers" are hot new supplements designed to shed pounds by preventing the absorption of fat. Several pharmaceutical companies are working to develop fat blockers as diet aids, but there are already several natural products being sold over the counter. One of them is chitosan, which is made from chitin, a substance found in the exoskeletons of shellfish such as shrimp and crabs. Like plant fiber, chitosan is not digested by the body. As chitosan passes through the digestive tract it can absorb four to six times its weight in fat, thereby flushing it out of the body before it can be metabolized and stored as excess pounds. The problem is that chitosan can also hamper the absorption of fat-soluble vitamins. In my opinion, this supplement should not be used for more than two weeks at a time.

Coenzyme-Q10

Co-Q10, which is essential for the production of energy in the body, is being promoted as a sports supplement on the grounds that anything necessary for energy is good for athletes. In reality, Co-Q10 is part of a complicated biochemical process that stimulates the mitochondria, the tiny powerhouses within the cells that produce adenosine triphosphate (ATP), the fuel that runs the body. Since Co-Q10 facilitates the production of energy, it may—at least indirectly—help burn calories that would normally be converted to fat. It is also a wonderful supplement for the heart and is routinely given to heart patients in Japan. However, unlike what some manufacturers would have you believe, taking a Co-Q10 supplement is not going to give you an energy surge. The usual dose is two 60-mg. capsules daily. (I prefer the gel form that has hawthorne extract, garlic, and cayenne added to the formula.)

Conjugated Linoleic Acid (CLA)

During a vigorous workout, your body pumps out anabolic hormones like testosterone and growth hormone that help build muscle. At the same time, however, you are also subjecting your body to stress, which will result in the production of catabolic, or muscle-wasting, hormones such as cortisol, which can counteract the effect of the muscle-building hormones. Conjugated linoleic acid (CLA) is a fatty acid that was originally used to fatten cattle and block the negative effect of stress hormones on livestock. When put to the test on humans by enterprising researchers, CLA was shown to reduce body fat while increasing muscle, which suggests that it may negate the effect of the muscle-wasting hormones. It may also be useful for people who want to lose weight. Muscle burns calories; therefore, the more muscle you have, the less likely you are to store excess calories as fat. Take three 600- to 1200-mg. capsules daily before meals.

Cordyceps

Cordyceps is derived from a Chinese mushroom that has traditionally been used to fight fatigue and promote vitality. It is now being marketed as a sports supplement. According to Chinese studies, cordyceps can also improve athletic performance and is widely used by Chinese athletes. It has long been used to treat asthma and respiratory problems, and researchers speculate that it may improve athletic performance by opening up the breathing passages, thereby allowing more oxygen into the body. Oxygen, critical for the production of energy by the cells, is essential for endurance. Cordyceps is sold alone or combined with other Chinese tonic herbs. Take two 525-mg. capsules daily with meals.

Creatine Monohydrate

Of all the sports supplements that have been marketed to date, creatine monohydrate is probably the most popular. Essential for the production of ATP, the fuel that runs the body, creatine is concentrated in skeletal muscles. Vigorous exercise depletes your muscles of their natural supply of creatine. Restoring creatine through supplements helps to reenergize tired muscle cells and increase stamina so that you can work out longer.

A study in the *International Journal of Sport Nutrition* has shown that people who take creatine supplements and exercise regularly lose more fat and develop better muscle tone than people who only work out and do not take creatine supplements.

Another study jointly performed by Texas Woman's University, the University of Texas Southwestern Medical Center, and the Cooper Clinic found that creatine enhanced the performance of male weight lifters, allowing them to lift heavier loads and do more repetitions.

Creatine is available as a powder, which can be mixed in water or juice, or as chewable wafers. Take 5000 mg. (1 tablespoon of powder) in juice or water daily.

Essential Fatty Acids

People who want to shed pounds or build muscle often follow very low-fat diets. On the surface, this makes sense because each gram of fat has twice the calories of protein or carbohydrate. Therefore, if you cut out the fat, you are theoretically producing more lean tissue or muscle.

But diets that are severely restricted in fat can actually have the opposite effect: they can ultimately cause you to gain fat and lose muscle, for several reasons. First, our bodies cannot function well without some fat. In fact, fat is necessary for the production of hormones (essential for the production of muscle) and the absorption of fat-soluble vitamins. In particular, we need essential fatty acids, a type of fat that our bodies cannot produce on their own. Second, if you don't eat some fat along with carbohydrates, you are liable to get hungrier faster, which will cause you to overeat. Carbohydrates trigger the release of the hormone insulin, which sends glycogen (sugar) into muscle cells. When the muscle cells are filled with glycogen, the excess is stored as fat. Combining a small amount of fat with carbohydrate can help slow down this process, giving your body more time to burn extra calories before they are converted to fat. Finally, a deficiency in essential fatty acids will result in some unpleasant symptoms, including very dry skin and hair.

If you are cutting down on calories, consider taking an essential fatty acid supplement. Flaxseed oil and borage oil (which is a bit pricier) are wonderful sources of essential fatty acids. You can add 1 to 2 tablespoons of oil to your food, or take 1 to 3 capsules daily.

Glycerol

When you exercise, it's important to replenish lost fluids. That is the principle behind glycerol, a new sports drink that helps the body retain water. Glycerol reputedly helps athletes hold onto fluid during vigorous exercise and to maintain a lower body temperature and a lower heart rate than can be achieved by merely drinking water. Sports supplements containing glycerol are available at sporting goods stores and natural food stores. Drink a glycerol sports drink 30 minutes before strenuous exercise, and immediately following exercise. Be sure to drink plenty of water while you exercise. If you are exercising for a long period of time—for example, running a marathon—you may need to replenish glycerol during the race.

Growth Hormone Boosters

L-arginine and L-glutamine are known for their ability to stimulate the production of growth hormone, which is instrumental in shedding fat and building muscle. As we age, our levels of growth hormone decline, which some experts believe is responsible for the muscle wasting that can lead to frailty among the elderly. The argument is that if the lack of growth hormone can cause muscle loss, then replenishing growth hormone should enhance muscle gain.

So why not just take growth hormone directly? Human growth hormone not only is very expensive (it can run up to $1000 a month) but is available by prescription only. In addition, growth hormone can cause some unpleasant side effects, including fluid retention and severe arthritis. Body builders are turning to natural growth hormone–releasing agents, such as L-arginine and L-glutamine, to bulk up and lose flab. It's interesting to note that vigorous exercise is a natural way to boost growth hormone, and some researchers believe that the benefits of exercise may actually be due to its ability to increase growth hormone production. In other words, if you exercise vigorously, you may not need to take growth hormone or growth hormone producing agents.

L-arginine and L-glutamine are often included in combination sports formulas.

Gymnema Sylvestre

This Ayurvedic herb may help you say no to sweets. Some people may find that drinking a cup of tea with a few drops of gymnema extract will make sweet things taste bitter for up to two hours afterwards. Try it and see if it works for you!

"Herbal Fen Phen"

As of this writing, "Fen Phen," the combination diet pill, has been recalled by its manufacturer because of reports of serious side effects among its users, such as potentially fatal heart valve problems. One alternative being offered is so-called herbal Fen Phen, a combination of a thermogenic enhancer (such as the herb ephedra) and the antidepressant Saint John's wort. It makes sense that these herbs would be helpful for losing weight. We know that ephedra can speed up metabolism, which helps the body burn fat faster. In addition, Saint John's wort is reputed to be a natural appetite suppressant. As yet, there are no studies to confirm that these herbs will work well together.

Beta-hydroxy Beta-methylbutyrate (HMB)

HMB is among the most popular of the new sports supplements. A byproduct of the breakdown in the body of an amino acid called leucine, HMB may enhance the effect of vigorous exercise by building muscle and reducing body fat. In one study conducted at Iowa State University, 40 men received either HMB supplements

(3 grams per day) or a placebo. All of the men underwent four weeks of weight training performed three days a week. At the end of the four weeks, the group taking the HMB showed a greater increase in muscle, lost more fat, and were stronger than those not taking HMB. You may get more from your workout by using this supplement. Take 3 grams daily in either capsule or powder form.

Hydroxycitrate (HCA or Garcinia)

Hydrocitric acid (HCA), also called garcinia, is a natural appetite suppressant and thermogenic agent that slows down the production of fat from the metabolism of carbohydrates and proteins. HCA enhances the ability of the liver and muscles to store glycogen, thereby reducing fat production and diminishing appetite. Animal studies have shown that HCA can suppress fat production by 40 to 80 percent for 8 to 12 hours after eating. Human studies have also confirmed that people eat less and store less body fat after taking HCA.

HCA is included in several weight-loss formulas, including diet drinks and bars. It is also available in capsules. Take up to three 500-mg. capsules before meals.

L-Carnitine

L-carnitine has been promoted as a sports supplement that can increase physical stamina and promote weight loss. In reality, studies have shown that L-carnitine can improve stamina and endurance during exercise for heart patients, but there is no solid evidence yet that it has any dramatic effect on healthy people. If you have a heart condition or suffer angina or chest pain during exercise, talk to your doctor about taking this supplement.

Pyruvate

This supplement is hot, new, and expensive. I'm not sure that it works at low doses (which can make it *very* pricey), but many body builders swear by it. Pyruvate, a natural substance found in the body, is critical for energy usage because it triggers the release of adenosine triphosphate (ATP), the fuel that runs the body. In a recent study, athletes who used pyruvate tired less easily and were able to increase their performance by an impressive 20 percent. Other studies show that people who are already following a low-calorie diet will lose even more weight if they take pyruvate.

As I mentioned earlier, the problem is that the only successful studies of pyruvate involved using 15 to 44 grams of pyruvate, which would run into a great deal of money (up to $13 daily at current prices!). Pyruvate's fans, of which there are many, contend that as little as 5 grams can achieve good results, which would significantly bring down the cost. Pyruvate is safe, and there are few side effects, except for occasional stomach upset. It also lowers cholesterol and blood pressure. You can try taking a low dose of pyruvate (5 grams per day) and see if it works for you.

Puncturevine

Also known as tribulus, this Ayurvedic herb is reputed to boost testosterone levels, which as I explained earlier may help build muscle and burn fat. Bulgarian studies showed that tribulus naturally increased the body's production of LH (luteinizing hormone), which stimulates the production of testosterone in men. Tribulus is popping up in many sports formulas combining different supplements primarily for men including DHEA and androstenedione.

When you use hormones, as I've also noted earlier, I recommend exercising some caution. Testosterone can be broken down into a more potent form, dihydrotestosterone, which can stimulate the growth of the prostate, causing benign prostate hypertrophy or the more serious prostate cancer. If you have a problem with your prostate or a family history of prostate cancer, I would avoid using testosterone-enhancing supplements.

Vanadyl Sulfate

In the words of my friend the body builder, vanadyl sulfate makes him feel "pumped." Vanadyl mimics the action of the hormone insulin, which regulates the metabolism of carbohydrate and protein, breaking them down into a form that can be utilized by the cells to make energy. Serious body builders swear that within two or three weeks of taking vanadyl sulfate they feel and see a real difference in the size and strength of their muscles. The problem with vanadyl is that it can cause a sudden drop in blood sugar, which can be dangerous. Do not use this supplement if you are hypoglycemic or suffer from diabetes unless you are under the care of a physician. For body building, the usual dose is 10 mg. half an hour before a workout.

Whey

Whey is a protein extracted from milk and is being promoted as the "perfect protein" for building strong muscles. Because of the high physical demand they place on themselves, body builders and athletes need additional protein to help maintain existing muscle and to build new muscle. Body builders consider whey protein concentrate to be the highest-quality form of protein because it is low in calories and fat and is easily absorbed by the body. Whey also contains powerful immune-enhancing compounds. Whey protein concentrate is sold by itself and is also included in numerous meal replacement powders. Dissolve 2 tablespoons (1 ounce) in half a cup of water or juice daily.

4

Mood-Enhancing Supplements

Coping with Depression Naturally

Depression is one of the most common medical problems in the West in general, and the United States in particular. About 17 million Americans suffer from depression at some point in their lives. Depression can be triggered by any number of factors, including a chemical imbalance or an emotionally upsetting event such as a divorce or a death in the family. The signs of depression include insomnia, loss of energy, change in appetite, feelings of sadness, and recurrent thoughts of death or suicide. If these or similar symptoms last for more than a week, you should seek medical advice—real depression is not a problem to be dismissed or taken lightly. Many people, however, suffer from a mild depression, or "the blues"—transitory feelings of sadness or unhappiness. These feelings may not interfere with normal functioning, but they can certainly hamper our ability to get the most out of life.

In recent years, the treatment of disorders such as depression and anxiety has been turned over to the pharmaceutical industry. As a result, millions of people are taking drugs like Prozac, Zoloft, and Paxil for depression, and Xanax and Valium for anxiety, often with unpleasant, unpredictable, or even dangerous side effects. The good news is that today there are some effective, safe, inexpensive natural alternatives to these drugs that can be purchased at natural food stores. In particular, these supplements are wonderful for people with mild depression who are reluctant to take prescription drugs but who can use a lift.

Before I describe these supplements, I don't want to suggest that all forms of depression can be "cured" simply by taking a pill. Eating sensibly, getting enough exercise, and living a life with spiritual sustenance are all important factors in maintaining a positive outlook on life. For instance, when I feel down, the first place I go is to the gym because I know that working out will help me feel better. Exercise boosts the production of endorphins, chemicals in the brain that can elevate mood. After a half hour or so on the treadmill, I can feel a difference. The second place I go is a magnificent nature preserve tucked away in the hills overlooking the Pacific Ocean. I find it is impossible to stay depressed when I am in such beautiful surroundings. When you feel down, try to find your own natural ways to get your spirits soaring. Very often, taking a few positive steps will help you feel better.

The following supplements can also help you shake the blues. If you are taking prescription antidepressants and want to switch to natural supplements, do not discontinue your prescription drugs without first consulting with your physician. In some cases, you may need to gradually reduce your dose to avoid withdrawal symptoms.

Are You Getting Enough B Vitamins?

B vitamins are especially important for normal brain function, and a deficiency in B vitamins (especially vitamin B_{12}) can result in symptoms such as depression, irritability, and apathy. About 10 percent of all people over 65 are deficient in vitamin B_{12}, which is found in meat, fish, eggs, and dairy products. As people age they may develop a condition called atrophic gastritis, meaning that they are producing less gastric acid, which hampers the ability of the body to utilize vitamin B_{12} in food.

Some people turn to alcohol when they are depressed, but this will only make matters worse, since alcohol can destroy B vitamins.

To make sure you are getting enough B vitamins, I recommend that you take the following: one 50-mg. vitamin B-complex capsule or tablet daily, one 500-mg. vitamin B_1 or thiamine capsule daily, and one 1000-mcg. vitamin B_{12} tablet in sublingual form (dissolved under the tongue).

Fish Eaters Are Happier

The connection between nutrition and mood is underscored by a recent study that links the increase in depression in Western countries to the decline in the consumption of cold-water fatty fish. These foods in general, and fatty fish in particular, are abundant in omega-3 fatty acids, which are essential for the proper functioning of many systems in the body and appear to be especially important for normal brain function.

Omega-3 fatty acids contain alpha-linolenic acid, which is metabolized into eicosapentaenoic acid (EPA) and docosahexaenoic acid (DHA) in the body. DHA is found in high concentration in the gray matter of the brain and the retina of the eye, and is instrumental in the function of brain cell membranes, which are important for the transmission of brain signals. Over the past 50 years, the consumption of omega-3 fatty acids has significantly declined in the West, and as a result we are ingesting less DHA. Instead, we are eating more omega-6 fatty acids, which are found in polyunsaturated oils and processed foods. In addition to reducing our intake of fish, we are not eating as many whole grains and seeds, which are also abundant in omega-3 fatty acids.

The overall decline in omega-3 consumption may be creating a DHA deficit that is damaging to our health in many different ways, especially our mental health. According to an article published in the *American Journal of Clinical Nutrition*, Dr. Joseph R. Hibbeln and Dr. Norman Salem of the National Institutes of Health have linked the increase in depression in North America over the past century to a steady decline in DHA consumption. The authors made this discovery while trying to solve a decade-old medical mystery. In 1984, a highly publicized study showed that when people were given a cholesterol-lowering diet, they suffered increased depression leading to suicide for reasons not fully understood. Scientists were further confounded by later studies that showed just the opposite to be true: when people were given heart-healthy diets, they were actually happier!

Why the contradictory results? After reviewing the studies, Drs. Hibbeln and Salem came to the startling conclusion that among the dieters, the people who lived near coastal regions where fresh fish was abundant were the happiest, and the people who lived inland where fresh fish was not as easy to find were the most depressed. In other words, depression was rare in regions where omega-3 consumption had remained high, but a common problem in areas where omega-3 consumption was low. Eating more fatty fish (such as salmon, sea bass, mackerel, albacore tuna, and sardines) is a good way to make sure that you are getting enough omega-3 fatty acids and DHA. Taking a supplement is another. DHA is also available in capsules; take three 250-mg. capsules daily.

The Natural Prozac: 5-HTP

Prozac belongs to a class of drugs known as selective serotonin reuptake inhibitors (SSRIs), which enhance the activity of serotonin, a hormone produced by the brain that is involved in mood, sleep, and appetite. Low levels of serotonin are associated with depression, anxiety, and sleep disorders. SSRIs prevent the brain cells from using up serotonin too quickly, thereby causing a deficiency. 5-Hydroxytryptophan (5-HTP) is a hot new supplement that does what the SSRIs cannot: increase the cells' production of serotonin to boost serotonin levels. When tested against standard SSRIs, 5-HTP has proved to be an equally effective antidepressant but without any of the negative side effects associated with SSRIs, such as dry mouth, reduced libido, heart palpitations, tremors, and anxiety. It is also a fraction of the cost and can be purchased without a prescription. In addition, 5-HTP has been used successfully to treat sleep disorders. Serotonin is the precursor to melatonin, the natural hormone that regulates sleep-wake cycles. When you boost your level of serotonin, you are also increasing your level of melatonin, which can result in a better night's sleep. Serotonin deficiency is also implicated in PMS, winter depression (also known as SAD), migraine headaches, anxiety, and violent behavior. Take two 50-mg. capsules daily.

Do not use 5-HTP with other antidepressants or mono-amine oxidase (MAO) inhibitors.

S-Adenosyl-L-Methione (SAMe)

SAMe is a natural substance produced by the body from methionine, an amino acid. SAMe is essential for many important functions in the body, from the production of protein to the manufacture of glutathione, the body's primary antioxidant. Recently, SAMe has been growing in popularity as a new antidepressant. I use the word "new" advisedly, because SAMe has been used in Europe for this purpose for more than 20 years. Literally hundreds of studies have been performed on SAMe, and it appears to be both safe and effective. Several studies have been devoted to the use of SAMe as an antidepressant for people suffering from depression alone, or depression induced by illnesses such as rheumatoid arthritis or Parkinson's disease. In study after study, SAMe performed well, even in comparison with prescription antidepressants. Unlike other pharmaceutic antidepressants that can cause dangerous side effects, such as liver damage and even cancer, SAMe can enhance overall health (see page 150). Most people can feel results in less than a week.

Take up to three 500-mg. capsules daily.

Saint John's Wort

Recently there has been a great deal of publicity about this herbal remedy for depression, which is the number-one antidepressant prescribed in Germany. Numerous studies have shown that Saint John's wort is both safe and effective. In fact, a recent study published in the *British Medical Journal* concluded that this herb worked as well as prescription antidepressants at a fraction of the cost, and without side effects. In fact, close to 70 million doses of this herb were prescribed in Germany in 1994, with virtually no reports of overdose, toxicity, negative drug interactions, or undue side effects.

The active ingredient in Saint John's wort is believed to be hypericum, which has also been used successfully to treat viral infections. It is currently being studied as a potential treatment for AIDS, hepatitis, cancer, arthritis, psoriasis, and ulcers. It is not fully understood how hypericum works. Researchers theorize that hypericum may block the binding of serotonin and other neurotransmitters, thereby preventing them from being used up too quickly. In addition, hypericum may inhibit the production of stress hormones that not only make us feel agitated but can dampen immune response.

Take up to three 250- to 500-mg. capsules daily. It may take up to eight weeks for you to feel any positive effects. Saint John's wort will increase photosensitivity—that is, make you more vulnerable to a sunburn. If you use this herb, stay out of the sun.

Tyrosine

Tyrosine, an amino acid, is the precursor to several important neurotransmitters in the brain that control mood, mental function, and even sex drive. It also plays an important role in the functioning of the adrenal, pituitary, and thyroid glands, which control hormone production in the body. People who are depressed often have low levels of tyrosine in the brain, and in fact, several prescription medications used to treat depression do so by boosting tyrosine levels.

Several studies have indicated that tyrosine supplements can be an effective treatment for depression and anxiety, without the side effects associated with antidepressants. Tyrosine also can help counteract the effect of stress. In one study, soldiers given tyrosine supplements performed better on mental tests, were more alert, had fewer complaints, and generally functioned at a higher level than those not given tyrosine. Natural healers prescribe tyrosine for women who suffer from PMS, and many find that it can reduce the fatigue, depression, and general feeling of discomfort often associated with this problem. Dopamine, which is critical for sex drive, is one of the neurotransmitters manufactured from tyrosine. In fact, tyrosine is often prescribed to rev up a sluggish libido. Not surprisingly, loss of sex drive is often a sign of depression. It is common for depressed people to lose interest not only in sex but in other life-affirming activities as well.

Although it has not been scientifically proven, some studies suggest that tyrosine may stimulate the production of growth hormone. If this turns out to be true, tyrosine may also help build muscle and reduce body fat. Tyrosine is also reputed to reduce appetite in some people. I suspect that tyrosine may not work directly on the appetite centers of the brain but rather may help uplift the spirits of those who turn to food for comfort when they are depressed.

Take two 500-mg. tablets or capsules twice daily, half an hour before eating.

Natural Stress Busters

The American Academy of Family Physicians recently released a study showing that two-thirds of all visits to family doctors result from stress-related ailments. Stress not only makes us feel tense and sapped of energy but also can have a profound effect on virtually every system of the body. Stress hormones—the hormones we produce when we are feeling keyed up—can raise blood pressure, inhibit the ability of the immune system to fight infection, raise blood sugar levels, promote osteoporosis, and even kill brain cells. For both your mental and physical health, it is important not to allow stress to overtake your life.

When we are under a great deal of stress, we may resort to destructive behaviors that only make matters worse. Drained of energy, we may use too much caffeine for a quick lift, only to find that the effects are very short-lived. In fact, excess intake of caffeine can exacerbate the symptoms of anxiety such as rapid heartbeat. Or we may try to calm down with prescription tranquilizers and sleeping pills, which may become addictive. There is a better way. Here are some wonderful natural remedies that can help reduce stress and anxiety, and help restore equilibrium.

Calcium and Magnesium

These two minerals, which are often missing from our diets, are natural stress busters that have a calming effect on the body. They can also lower blood pressure. Take a combination tablet with 500 mg. of calcium and 250 mg. of magnesium.

Kava Kava

For 3,000 years, residents of the South Pacific have used a beverage made from the herb kava kava, a member of the pepper family, to induce a feeling of well-being and relaxation. That's why I always chuckle when I see kava kava being promoted as the cutting-edge, "new" herb for anxiety—it's only new to us. Just recently scientists verified what Polynesians have known for centuries: kava kava is a natural mood enhancer. In 1993, scientists discovered that kava kava contains potent compounds, kavalactones, which are natural muscle relaxants that have a pleasant, calming effect on both the body and the mind. Several studies have shown that kavalactones can reduce the symptoms of anxiety as well as or even better than prescription antianxiety drugs, but without the unpleasant side effects such as dry mouth and nausea. Even better, kava kava is nonaddictive and will not leave you feeling drugged or groggy, as do many tranquilizers. You should feel calm yet alert.

Recently, I encountered a new and interesting use for kava kava as a treatment for the symptoms of menopause. In one study, a group of 20 postmenopausal women were given either kava kava supplements daily or a placebo. The group taking kava kava experienced an almost immediate improvement in symptoms of stress, anxiety, and even hot flashes.

Take up to three 250-mg. capsules daily. Do not exceed the recommended dosage.

Caution

Although kava kava will not make most people drowsy, there is a small risk that it may. When you first begin taking kava kava, closely monitor your reaction to this herb. If you feel drowsy or "out of it" after taking kava kava, don't drive or engage in any activity that requires concentration.

Calm Down with Flower Essences

Flower essences are homeopathic-type liquid dilutions prepared from the essences of several flowers that are reputed to relieve stress, depression, and anxiety. The most famous, Rescue Remedy, was developed in the 1930s by Edward Bach, who believed that flowers possessed unique "vibrational energy" that could soothe the human spirit. A more scientific explanation is that the faint scent emitted by the flowers may affect brain chemistry. Flower essences, which are sold in natural food stores, are very easy to use and completely nontoxic. Many people find the experience to be quite relaxing. Simply put a few drops of the liquid essence under your tongue, or add a few drops to your beverage of choice and sip slowly.

DHEA: Reduce Stress and Boost Your Spirits

This Hot 100 supplement is a natural hormone that declines as we age. DHEA is a natural mood enhancer that appears to have a significant effect on our emotional well-being. People who take DHEA—myself included— notice that it can relieve stress and boost mood. A primary role of DHEA in the body is to control the action of stress hormones. In one study, rats were given a large dose of a chemical that mimics the effect of stress hormones in the body and sends blood pressure soaring. Ultimately, the rats died. Amazingly, if the rats were given DHEA before being given the lethal drug, they survived and their blood pressure remained normal.

In a recent study conducted at the University of San Diego, DHEA supplements were given to 13 men and 17 women, aged 40 to 70, for three months, and a placebo for three months. During the time they were taking the DHEA, the researchers reported that the volunteers felt happier and stronger and said they were better able to cope with stress.

Even though DHEA is sold over the counter, it is still wise to have your DHEA levels checked by your doctor to see whether you need to take this supplement. DHEA is not necessary for most people under 40, since the body is probably making enough. But people in their mid-40s and beyond will probably find that they are low in DHEA. The usual dose is up to two 25-mg. tablets daily for men and one 25-mg. tablet daily for women. For best results, take DHEA in the morning. (For more information on DHEA, see page 49.)

Aromatherapy

Numerous studies have shown the power of essential oils to induce relaxation, reduce anxiety, and ease depression. Essential oils stimulate the olfactory organs, which are linked to the areas of the brain that control emotions. Simply rub a few drops of essential oil on your skin, or put a few drops of essential oil in a diffuser to scent the room. Use essential oils at home or at work. Essential oils should *never* be ingested.

Lavender Oil

For more than a thousand years, herbalists have recommended lavender to treat stress and related conditions such as insomnia. Recent studies suggest that it does indeed have a soothing effect on the body. Recently, researchers in England tested whether lavender oil could be used as a treatment for insomnia for nursing home residents. Four patients who had been receiving sleep medication for up to three years had their sleep measured for six weeks. For the first two weeks, the medication was tapered off. The second two weeks, the patients were given no medication. The last two weeks, the patients did not get any medication, and their rooms were perfumed with lavender oil. Researchers found that the patients had difficulty sleeping during the second two weeks when their medication was discontinued, but amazingly, during the last two weeks, they slept as well with the lavender oil as they had with their medication.

Citrus Oil

According to a recent Japanese study, citrus oil combined with antidepressants helped patients suffering from chronic depression. Ten patients were regularly exposed to a citrus-based perfume developed by Shiseido, in addition to taking more than 100 mg. of antidepressants daily. By the end of 11 weeks, all but one patient was able to stop taking the antidepressants as long as they continued their aromatherapy.

Valerian

Known as "herbal Valium," this herb is used to treat insomnia, stress, and tension headaches. (Despite its name, it is completely unrelated to the synthetic drug Valium.) Numerous studies have confirmed that valerian is an effective aid to sleep. It is also excellent for muscle spasms, which are often caused by stress. This herb is safe and not habit-forming, but it doesn't work for everybody. In rare cases, it can have the opposite effect and be too stimulating. Valerian is available in extracts, capsules, and tablets. Try one capsule; if it makes you feel relaxed, then you know it works for you. Since valerian can cause sleepiness, use it only at night.

Siberian Ginseng

A relative of Asian ginseng, Siberian ginseng is a tonic herb that helps protect the body against the ill effects of stress. This herb not only helps us better cope with nervous tension but at the same time increases stamina and mental alertness. For decades, the Russians have been giving Siberian ginseng to athletes to help build their endurance. If you think about it, this makes perfect sense. Athletic competition can be very stressful on all systems of the body, which will cause athletes to fatigue more easily. Take up to three 500-mg. capsules a half hour before eating. Although Siberian ginseng can lower moderately high blood pressure, it may have the opposite effect on very high blood pressure. If you are being treated for high blood pressure, do not use this herb.

5

Super Hot Supplements to Jump-Start Your Sex Life

Since the beginning of time, natural healers have searched for the ultimate aphrodisiac: a pill or potion that could not only enhance sexual desire but guarantee a stellar performance. Every culture has its share of remedies that are supposed to rev up sex drive and improve sexual function. At one time, "modern thinkers" dismissed these claims as ridiculous. In fact, until recently, it was assumed that sexual complaints were primarily psychological problems, but we now know that many of these problems are rooted in poor physical health.

Ancient healers were surprisingly sophisticated in that many so-called aphrodisiacs were actually designed to treat physical conditions that were the underlying cause of sexual dysfunction. If fatigue was sapping your interest in sex, tonics such as ginseng or ashwagandha were prescribed for stamina and energy. If a sluggish libido was creating friction between spouses, herbs such as tribulus, muira puama, and sarsaparilla were recommended to boost hormone levels for both sexes. If atherosclerosis (blockage of the arteries) was making it impossible for a man to sustain an erection, herbs such as ginkgo biloba or yohimbe were prescribed to increase blood flow to the penis. It took us centuries to discover what these healers knew intuitively: Good health is the best aphrodisiac of all.

Before describing how supplements can enhance sex, I want to make one point. Maintaining a strong, well-functioning body is the best way to maintain a satisfying sex life. Eating the right foods and living a healthy lifestyle will keep your body and mind in great shape. Destructive habits such as smoking, alcohol abuse, or a diet laden with sugar and "bad" fat will inevitably create the types of physical problems that will destroy your sex life. In fact, it may surprise you to learn that more than half of all potency problems in men are actually caused by poor circulation due to atherosclerosis—a problem that's directly related to heart disease, not reproductive function. Atherosclerosis can block blood flow to the penis, making it difficult to have or maintain an erection. In addition, atherosclerosis increases the odds of developing diabetes, which can cause nerve damage that can hamper the ability to feel sensation. Although the most common sexual problems in women are caused by discomfort due to menopause, women are also susceptible to atherosclerosis, which may not interfere directly with sexual function but can sap them of the vitality and energy needed for satisfying sex. To compound these problems, many of the prescription medications routinely prescribed to treat conditions such as diabetes, atherosclerosis, and high blood pressure can also cause side effects that include loss of sex drive and impotence. (Even commonly used drugs such as antacids and antidepressants can dampen sexual response.)

Most of the problems that wreak havoc on our sex

lives can be prevented or even reversed through the right combination of diet, exercise, and supplements.

It may also surprise you to know that the more active your lifestyle, the more active your sex life. According to one study of 160 master swimmers between the ages of 40 and 80, men who exercised the most had sex lives typical of people 20 to 30 years their junior. But you don't have to be a career athlete to enjoy the benefits of better sex. In another study, 78 previously sedentary but healthy men began a moderate exercise program in which they either jogged or rode their bikes for an hour every other day. A control group of 17 men did not exercise. After nine months, the exercisers reported a 30 percent increase in sexual activity and a 26 percent increase in frequency of orgasm!

Taking the right supplements is another way to enhance your sex life. Supplements not only can prevent many of the problems that interfere with normal sexual function but can stimulate sexual desire and even improve performance. So get out your running shoes, jog to your natural food store, and check out these supersexy supplements.

Vitamin A

This fat-soluble vitamin is essential for the production of hormones for both sexes. If your diet is very low in fat, you are probably not getting enough vitamin A. Take one 5000-IU capsule daily.

L-Arginine

This Hot 100 amino acid is involved in nitric oxide production, which is essential for erections. Men who use it report that they have stronger and longer-lasting erections. (For more information, see page 3.) For best results, take 3 to 6 grams of L-arginine on an empty stomach 45 minutes before having sex.

Astralagus

This herb is used in China as a tonic to revitalize, strengthen, and restore sexual energy and physical endurance in men and women. Astralagus can also boost immune function and overall general health. This herb may also be useful to treat male infertility due to poor sperm motility, which makes it difficult for conception to occur. In one test tube study, astralagus improved sperm motility, which suggests it would work as well in human beings.

Take up to three 400-mg. capsules daily.

Avena Sativa

You've heard the expression "Sow your wild oats." Whoever first coined that phrase must have had avena sativa in mind. Derived from the wild oat plant, avena sativa is reputed to increase libido in both men and women. Preliminary studies conducted on a small group of men and women at the Institute for Advanced Human Sexuality in San Francisco showed that this herb raised the level of free testosterone (unbound, available testosterone) in men. This is important, because as men age, their level of free testosterone declines, and this can reduce their sex drive and hamper performance. Although few clinical studies have been performed on avena sativa, a wealth of anecdotal reports indicates that it really works. Users claim that it not only stimulates interest in sex but enables more and better orgasms. Try it and see if it works for you.

Take up to three capsules daily.

Caffeine

We use caffeine so often that we don't even think of it as a supplement, but it *is* strong medicine. Caffeinated beverages (coffee, tea, and cola drinks) provide an immediate lift that increases energy and stamina. Caffeine may also increase sex drive. According to a survey at the University of Michigan of 2,000 people over the age of 60, those who drank at least one cup of coffee daily had more sexual activity than non–coffee drinkers. The researchers speculated that the stimulating effect of caffeine in the coffee could be why the coffee drinkers were sexier! If you indulge in caffeine, don't overdo it. Stick to one or two cups daily, preferably early in the day, long before you go to sleep. Too much caffeine can cause heart palpitations and fatigue. Be sure to steer clear of caffeine pills and tablets—these products can produce adverse effects in some people.

Cayenne Pepper

This "hot" herb can heat up your sex life! Cayenne pepper contains capsaicin, which helps to raise metabolism and stimulate circulation. Increasing metabolism will help burn fat faster, which will enhance energy production for both men and women. The more energetic you feel, the more likely you are to feel romantic. In addition, cayenne can help control high blood cholesterol levels, which can lead to atherosclerosis, the number-one cause of male sex problems.

Take up to three 500-mg. capsules daily.

Damiana

Highly regarded as an aphrodisiac in Central America, damiana is used by both men and women to maintain sexual health. Because of its balancing effect on hormones, damiana is often prescribed for women to treat PMS and menopausal symptoms. Historically, damiana has been given to men as a treatment for premature ejaculation and urinary tract infections. Damiana's reputation as a sex-enhancing supplement may be due to the fact of its mildly stimulant properties, which enhance feelings of alertness and energy. Some herbalists believe that damiana slightly irritates the urethra in men, thus sensitizing the penis and making it more responsive to stimulation.

Take one 60-mg. capsule up to three times daily.

DHEA

Men report that this natural hormone makes them feel stronger and sexier. This makes sense; DHEA is broken down into testosterone in the body, which will have a definite effect on libido. DHEA's effect on male sexuality was documented in the Massachusetts Male Aging Study, in which researchers investigated, among other things, sexual activity in men ages 40 to 70. On the basis of this study, at least half of all men experience occasional impotence—that is, difficulty maintaining an erection. Interestingly, the men most likely to suffer from impotence were those with the lowest levels of DHEA. Cigarette smoking and excess alcohol consumption also greatly increased the odds of male impotence.

DHEA is also a natural energizer and antidepressant for both sexes. A recent Canadian study showed that

DHEA can be effective in relieving menopausal symptoms in women.

The usual dose is 50 mg. daily for men over 40 and 25 mg. daily for women over 40. Take DHEA in the morning for best absorption.

Dong Quai

If common menopausal symptoms, such as hot flashes, vaginal dryness, and excessive fatigue, are decreasing your libido, this herb may be the answer. Long used in Asia as a treatment for menopause, dong quai contains natural plant estrogens that can relieve menopausal symptoms and restore energy. Dong quai is also a wonderful antidote for stress.

Take up to three 500-mg. capsules daily.

Ginkgo Biloba

Ginkgo biloba is the herb for good circulation, and good circulation is essential for good sex. It's as simple as that. Studies have shown that ginkgo can be an effective treatment for erection problems caused by inadequate blood flow. Every man who wants to stay sexually fit should take this herb!

Take up to three 60-mg. capsules or tablets of standardized ginkgo daily.

Fertilized Chicken Eggs

According to an old wives' tale, if you crack open a fertilized chicken egg, it means that the stork will soon be paying you a visit. This may not be as silly as it sounds. A supplement derived from fertilized chicken eggs, marketed under the names of Libido and Virilite, has been used successfully in Europe to treat problems associated with low sex drive. As of this writing, these products are very new to the United States and should be arriving shortly.

For best results, follow the directions on the package.

Ginseng

In Asia, ginseng remains the most popular herb for restoring sexual desire and function. Best known as a tonic herb that can improve overall health, ginseng is also a rich source of plant hormones, which can enhance both energy levels and sex drive. Although human studies are scarce, animal studies have shown that ginseng can increase testosterone levels, sperm production, and sexual activity in males. Because it is such a rich source of plant hormones, menopausal women use ginseng to relieve menopausal symptoms. (For more information, see page 184.)

Take up to six 500-mg. capsules daily.

Muira Puama

Native to Brazil, this herb is also called "potency wood." According to a recent study conducted at the Institute of Sexology in Paris, it may live up to its reputation. In the study, 262 men who complained of low sex drive or erection problems were given 1 to 1.5 grams of muira extract daily. About 60 percent of the men reported feeling positive effects within two weeks, especially men who had reported having difficulty maintaining an erection. Muira puama is included in male potency formulas sold at natural food stores.

Natural Progesterone Cream

This Hot 100 supplement is known as the "feel-good" hormone for women because it improves mood and enhances sex drive. Progesterone levels are higher during pregnancy, a time when many women experience a sense of euphoria. In addition, they are highest during the time in the menstrual cycle when women are the most fertile and when they often experience an increase in sex drive. After menopause, progesterone production slows down. Studies and numerous anecdotal accounts confirm that replenishing lost progesterone can make a woman feel happier, healthier, and sexier.

Use ¼ to ½ teaspoon of progesterone cream twice daily on abdomen, inner thighs, arms, or face.

Niacin (Vitamin B₃)

What's this mainstream B vitamin doing on my list of sexy supplements? Niacin is the vitamin that helps keep blood flowing freely throughout the body by dilating blood vessels. In the Hot 100, I recommend a "non-flush" form of niacin called inositol hexanicotinate to help lower elevated blood cholesterol levels. According to John Morgenthaler's book *Better Sex Through Chemistry*, niacin can also stimulate the release of a histamine that is necessary for orgasm.

Take up to three 500-mg. tablets daily. (Inositol hexanicotinate does not cause flushing, redness, or itchiness typical of other forms of niacin.)

Sarsaparilla

After a long cattle drive, cowboys in the know would bypass their local saloons and head over to the general merchandise store, where they would stock up on sarsaparilla, a popular beverage in the Wild West. Why? Long touted as an aphrodisiac, sarsaparilla is reputed to boost testosterone levels—the cowboys who drank it swore that it enhanced their sexual performance. Undoubtedly, what also helped was the fact that these guys weren't guzzling down whiskey, since alcohol can lower testosterone levels and inhibit sexual performance.

Take up to three capsules daily.

Yohimbe

This Hot 100 herb is a traditional treatment for male potency problems. It is sold alone or included in male potency formulas. When combined with zinc, ginkgo biloba, and L-arginine, yohimbe works well for many men. Yohimbe is not for everyone, however, and for some men, it may be dangerous. Be sure to read the information beginning on page 174 before using yohimbe.

Zinc

Semen contains high concentrations of zinc along with vitamin E, fructose, glucose, citric acid, selenium, proteins, and enzymes. Low levels of zinc have been associated with a sluggish sex drive and infertility in men. Zinc is also the most abundant mineral in the prostate, a small walnut-shaped gland under the urethra that can become enlarged as men age and cause great discomfort. Marginal zinc deficiency is very common among older men in the United States. Take one 15-mg. tablet daily.

6

A Brief Guide to Homeopathy

Homeopathy has been called New Age medicine, but in reality, it is based on principles that are more than 2,000 years old. Hippocrates, the Greek physician known as the father of medicine, once said, "Look for the cure in the cause." In a nutshell, that is the philosophy of modern homeopathy.

The word *homeopathy* tells the story: *homeos* means "similar," and *pathos* means "suffering." The underlying principle of homeopathy is very simple. Symptoms of an illness are signs that the body is trying to heal itself. Instead of attempting to suppress these symptoms with drugs, as is the practice in conventional medicine, the goal of homeopathy is to allow the symptoms to express themselves fully, thereby turning on the body's own healing powers.

Modern homeopathy was founded about 200 years ago by Samuel Hahnemann, a well-known German physician who was seeking an alternative to the often dangerous and ineffective methods used by his colleagues. Concerned about the common medical practices of the day, which included the indiscriminate use of poisonous mercury-based laxatives and blood-letting, Dr. Hahnemann believed that there must be a better way to treat patients. Intrigued by Hippocrates' writings on illness, Dr. Hahnemann performed a now famous experiment in which he ate cinchona bark, a well-known folk cure for malaria. After ingesting the bark, Dr. Hahnemann developed high fevers that were similar to the symptoms of malaria itself. As soon as he stopped taking the cinchona, the symptoms disappeared. Dr. Hahnemann intuitively reasoned that if a large dose of cinchona created malaria-like symptoms in a healthy person, perhaps a very small dose taken by a person who already had malaria could stimulate the body to cure the disease on its own. After years of experimentation, Dr. Hahnemann developed his theory, "Like cures like," also known as the Law of Similars. In other words, substances that in large doses can make healthy people sick, in small doses can help bring about a cure. If the Law of Similars sounds familiar, it is because it resembles the theory behind vaccines—that is, the practice of using a minute quantity of a virus to stimulate the body to produce antibodies against a particular disease.

Dr. Hahnemann spent years testing the effects of different medicines on healthy people, a process he called "provings." His work is described in his book *Chronic Diseases: Their Nature and Homeopathy Cure,* which revolutionized the practice of medicine. What is particularly intriguing is that several decades before Sigmund Freud's work, Dr. Hahnemann recognized that mental state played a role in illness.

Homeopathic preparations are very dilute forms of substances that if taken in large doses create symptoms similar to those of the illness that the remedy is meant to treat. For example, as most people know, large doses of ipecac can cause vomiting and stomach upset. Yet, a very dilute form of homeopathic ipecac is used to treat these very symptoms.

The potency of a homeopathic remedy is in inverse proportion to the amount of dilutions. So, for example, a homeopathic preparation identified as 10,000X means that it has been diluted 10-fold, four times. On the basis of this reasoning, a 10-fold dilution is stronger than a 2-, 4-, or 6-fold dilution. In other words, less is more. According to homeopathic theory, when a substance is diluted, it is potentized.

In the nineteenth century, homeopathy became very popular throughout Europe and the United States. Homeopathy has had some great success stories. For example, during a yellow fever epidemic in New Orleans in 1879, the mortality rate of patients treated by homeopathic physicians was 5.6 percent, whereas conventional physicians lost 16 percent of their patients. Homeopathic physicians were also quite adept at treating cholera and achieved a much higher survival rate than reported by conventional physicians. At the turn of the century, many American medical doctors also practiced homeopathic medicine, but homeopathy fell out of favor when the focus of medicine shifted to the use of antibiotics and other drugs. In Europe, homeopathy is still practiced alongside conventional medicine. In fact, members of the British royal family are treated by homeopathic physicians. In recent years, there has been a resurgence in interest in homeopathy in the United States, as with other forms of alternative medicine.

Traditional homeopathy is practiced by homeopathic physicians or healers who develop a custom-made preparation for each patient, which may be administered only in a single dose. In traditional homeopathy, the healer sits down and talks with the patient for an hour or more, and then, going by the patient's symptoms and personality, develops a remedy uniquely suited to that patient. This process is called repertorization. The goal is not just to treat the illness, but to find a remedy that resonates with each patient's "vital force," or inner energy. The choice of remedy is determined not only by symptom but by the patient's personality and demeanor. For example, a person with a headache who is sad and weepy is prescribed a different remedy from someone who has a headache but is irritable and agitated. In many respects, the traditional homeopathic practitioner is part healer, part psychologist.

Contemporary homeopathy, as its name suggests, is a more modern approach to this 200-year-old system of healing. It is no longer necessary to go to a homeopathic practitioner to obtain a homeopathic remedy; there are now numerous homeopathic preparations sold in natural food stores and pharmacies. Nor do you need to know much about homeopathy to use them; like other over-the-counter preparations, homeopathic products are clearly labeled. You use them in much the same way as other over-the-counter medications, and for the same problems. For instance, you might consider taking a homeopathic remedy for a cold, flu, headache, indigestion, or insomnia. However, if you do not feel better within 24 hours, or the symptoms worsen, it is a sign that you should call your physician or natural healer. Because homeopathic remedies are so diluted, there are no side effects from homeopathy.

The big question is this: can any remedy that is diluted down to the point where it is barely detectable actually be effective? There is a great deal of skepticism among some scientists that homeopathy works at all. Yet, several well-run studies have recently shown that homeopathic preparations are effective for many problems. In one famous study conducted in Nicaragua and published in *Pediatrics*, American physician Jennifer Jacobs tested a homeopathic remedy for diarrhea on children, 6 months to 5 years old, in a double-blind, placebo-controlled study. The children who received the homeopathic preparation recovered significantly faster (within five days) than those given the placebo. Studies published in the *British Medical Journal* and *Lancet* have confirmed that homeopathy has been helpful for rheumatoid arthritis, headaches, gastrointestinal problems, ankle sprains, and other problems that are often treated with over-the-counter medicines. Scientists have struggled to try to explain why homeopathy works, and the theories are fascinating. One theory is based on the work of a German biophysicist who through using highly sophisticated techniques such as magnetic resonance imaging (MRI) showed that homeopathic remedies emit measurable electromagnetic signals that are unique to each substance. So even though the remedy is so dilute that the original cure is undetectable, it may be working on a deeper, molecular level within the body.

It has been estimated that about 500 million people worldwide use homeopathic treatments. In France, Oscillococcinum, a homeopathic product that is gaining popularity in the United States, is the biggest selling over-the-counter cold and flu remedy.

There are more than 2,000 homeopathic preparations. Although many homeopathic products utilize herbs, homeopathic medicine is different from other herbal treatments in that homeopathic doses are potentized (diluted). Homeopathic remedies are under FDA regulation and must adhere to the same manufacturing practices as pharmaceutical companies. Unlike FDA-approved drugs, however, homeopathic remedies are not required to undergo the same expensive and arduous approval process. The following are some of the most commonly used homeopathic remedies. Most prepackaged products include a combination of several different homeopathic remedies. For example, a product designed to treat the flu might include several different remedies for respiratory ailments, coughs, headache, and body ache.

Aconitum

Also known as monkshood, this remedy is included in formulas to be taken at the first sign of a cold, flu, or ear infection. Signs that you need aconitum include the quick onset of a scratchy throat or chills. This remedy is also prescribed for insomnia due to emotional upset or fear.

Allium Cepa

What happens when you cut an onion? Your eyes get teary and your nose gets stuffy, almost as if you have a cold. In keeping with the principle that "like cures like," this homeopathic remedy made from red onion is used to treat sloppy colds, allergic reactions, and hay fever.

Arnica

Arnica is used to treat bruises, sprains, and muscle strains. Homeopathic ointment can be rubbed directly on the affected area. Although arnica ordinarily should not be ingested, homeopathic arnica is safe and can be taken to relieve pain. Do not apply arnica to broken or bleeding skin.

Arsenicum Album

A poison can also be a homeopathic remedy; such is the case with arsenic. In high doses, arsenic can cause death from poisoning, but in homeopathic doses, it is used to treat diarrhea, vomiting, stomach pain, and even food poisoning. Interestingly, arsenic is a traditional remedy for inflammatory skin conditions such as psoriasis.

Belladonna

Also known as deadly nightshade, this remedy shows up in homeopathic preparations designed to treat high fevers, bad colds, sore throats, headache, and painful ear infections. Interestingly, homeopathic practitioners recommend belladonna when the pain from an ear infection is more severe in the right ear. According to homeopathic orthodoxy, people who respond well to belladonna are very sensitive to light.

Bryonia

This is a popular remedy for dry coughs that are made worse by exposure to warmth or movement. In addition, bryonia is recommended for tension headaches that are exacerbated by movement or that cause throbbing pain on the right side of the head. Traditional homeopathic practitioners might use bryonia on revved-up Type A personalities who are consumed with work and are often edgy and irritable.

Calendula

A homeopathic ointment made of calendula and other herbs (such as comfrey, arnica, or bee propolis) may be used on minor cuts and wounds. Calendula can help fight infection and speed healing.

Carbo Vegetabilis

If you're gassy no matter what you eat, and feel better after belching, this remedy is for you.

Chamomilla

Chamomilla is used in formulas designed to treat severe headache, insomnia, or indigestion. It is also recommended for menstrual cramps and for teething pain in babies.

Coffee

Are you too excited to sleep? A remedy made from unroasted coffee is used to treat insomnia due to over-stimulation or excitement.

Colocynthis

Also known as bitter cucumber, this remedy can help soothe a colicky, upset stomach.

Euphrasia

This remedy is used to treat the earliest stages of a cold and allergies. It is recommended when the mucus discharge is clear (as opposed to allium cepa, which is to be used when the discharge is thick and heavy.) Homeopathic healers say it is especially good for watery, itchy eyes.

Ferrum Phosphoricum

Also called iron phosphate, this remedy is recommended to treat moderately high fever (about 102° F), sore throat, and swollen tonsils.

Gelsemium

Gelsemium is recommended for a dull headache and insomnia, especially when the inability to sleep is due to anxiety about the next day, or to stage fright. If you're up at night worrying about taking a big test in the morning or making a presentation at work, try this remedy.

Ignatia

Dubbed the "homeopathic Prozac," ignatia is recommended for people suffering from grief, emotional tumult, or anxiety-related problems such as depression, insomnia, or gastric upset due to stress. Ignatia has a calming effect on the body.

Lycopodium

Also known as club moss, this remedy is prescribed for a sore throat that feels better after a warm drink, for a gassy stomach, and for performance anxiety. The person who needs lycopodium is one who tries to mask his or her lack of self-confidence with bluster and bravado.

Nux Vomica

This is the most popular remedy for nausea and stomach upset due to excess imbibing. Nux vomica, also known as poison nut, contains tiny amounts of the poison strychnine. Homeopathic practitioners also prescribe this remedy to agitated, irritable, competitive people who suffer from chronic heartburn.

Pulsatilla

If you suffer from PMS, menstrual pain, or menopausal mood swings, this remedy is recommended to help you restore balance. It may be taken when you feel clingy or emotional. It is also included in products designed to relieve colic in infants.

Rhus Toxicodendron

Better known as poison ivy, this remedy is recommended for arthritis or sports injuries. People who are extremely agitated or restless may benefit from remedies that include rhus toxicodendron. It is also used to relieve the symptoms of shingles and chicken pox.

Sarsaparilla

This remedy is routinely prescribed for bladder infections, whose symptoms include burning or pain during urination. (Bladder infections can be serious and lead to kidney problems. Be sure to check with your physician or natural healer before self-medicating.)

Veratrum Album

If you are vomiting, have diarrhea, or suffer from nausea, and feel weak, this remedy may help. Homeopathic healers say that this remedy is indicated if you crave cold water and then vomit immediately after drinking it.

7

Hot Supplements from Around the World

Westerners like to believe that we invented the practice of medicine, but in fact, with a mere 200 or so years of experience under our belts, our medical system is very much the new kid on the block. Thousands of years before the invention of medical schools and pharmacies, there were shamans and healers practicing their own brands of traditional medicine with remarkable success. In many parts of the world today, they still are. Unlike Western medicine, which is primarily a "sick-care" system that focuses on curing illness, traditional systems of medicine emphasize wellness. It is the job of the healer to prevent illness from occurring in the first place.

Although we barely acknowledge their existence, we owe an enormous debt to the practitioners of traditional medicine. It may surprise you to learn that at least half of all pharmaceutical drugs used in the West—including many of our most successful cancer drugs—are derived from herbs and supplements used by ancient healers.

As Westerners turn to alternative medicine, there is a renewed interest in the concept of preventive medicine and the use of supplements to maintain health and vitality. In this section, I will describe some of the traditional systems of medicine and also review some of the "new" supplements appearing in natural food stores that are commonly used throughout the world.

Ayurvedic Medicine

More than 6,000 years old, India's Ayurvedic system of medicine is the oldest recorded medical system in the world, with ancient medical writings dating back to about 4500 B.C. It is still practiced in India today. *Ayurveda* is a Sanskrit word derived from two words, *ayur*, which means "life," and *veda*, which means "knowledge." Ayurvedic medicine has been dubbed the "mother of all healing" because of the profound influence it has had on nearly every other medical system practiced in both hemispheres. Early writings show that Ayurvedic practitioners were light-years ahead of their time in their knowledge of the powerful healing properties of plants. In this respect, they are the founders of modern pharmacology. They also had a sophisticated knowledge of the workings of the body, and there is even evidence that Ayurvedic physicians performed surgery. Diet and spirituality were and still are equally important parts of Ayurvedic medicine. The concepts of Ayurveda were spread by Buddhist monks who opened monasteries throughout the East, where each culture adapted those basic principles to accommodate its own national personality and beliefs. The traditional Chinese system of medicine, as well as much of the medicine practiced by Hippocrates, known as the father of modern medicine, has its roots in Ayurvedic medicine.

The underlying philosophy behind Ayurveda is that it is not enough to treat the symptoms of disease—

treatment must encompass the entire body. For example, an Ayurvedic healer would not simply prescribe an herb to treat the illness but would develop an entire program for the patient, including a food plan and lifestyle changes. It's ironic to note that in the West, we call this approach complementary medicine, and the physicians who practice it are considered novel and "cutting-edge." In reality, it's as old as recorded history.

There are many lessons to be learned from Ayurvedic medicine, but the most important of all may be that early intervention can make a real difference in the lives of patients. An example is the Ayurvedic approach to menopause. In the West, menopause is not usually treated until women begin experiencing telltale symptoms such as hot flashes, and only then are synthetic hormones prescribed to reduce their symptoms, often with potentially dangerous side effects. According to Philip Duterme, president of Ayurvedic Concepts, a new line of standardized Ayurvedic supplements, Indian women do not wait until menopause to deal with hormonal changes; they anticipate them years ahead of time. Starting at about the age of 20, women typically use herbal preparations to help normalize hormone levels throughout their lives, to ease the monthly hormonal fluctuations that can lead to PMS, and ultimately to ease the transition from the reproductive years to menopause. As a result, these women do not experience the abrupt drop in hormones that can cause severe menopausal symptoms.

Growing in popularity by leaps and bounds, numerous Ayurvedic products are being sold in natural food stores today. Although some herbs are sold individually, in traditional Ayurvedic medicine, herbs are used only in combination with other herbs. In addition, Ayurvedic practitioners frown on the Western concept that it is far better to extract the one or two active ingredients in an herb than to use the entire plant. Ayurvedic healers use the whole plant because they believe that every chemical in a plant is designed to work in harmony in the body. Rather than look for the magic bullet that will affect one key bodily function, Ayurvedic medicine is designed to bolster and support all body systems.

More than 2,000 different preparations are used in Ayurvedic medicine. Many include some of the most popular herbs in the world, such as garlic, aloe, ginger, and turmeric. Others are more exotic. The following is a description of some of the most widely used Ayurvedic herbal preparations that are available in natural food stores. Several have already been listed in the Hot 100, but here I will describe their traditional uses as opposed to how these herbs are being marketed for Western consumption. Ayurvedic herbs are typically sold in combination formulas; therefore, I do not give an individual dose for each herb. Follow the package directions.

Amalaki

The richest-known plant source of vitamin C (containing 3000 mg. per fruit), amalaki is a potent antioxidant. It is included in Ayurvedic formulas to boost immune function and to treat colds and coughs. It is also reputed to build and maintain bone, probably because vitamin C can stimulate the growth of collagen. Amalaki is also prescribed to treat vision problems.

Ashwagandha

The fundamental difference between Ayurvedic and Western medicine is underscored by the Ayurvedic use of tonics, herbs that are used not to treat specific ailments but to maintain overall health and vitality. Ashwagandha is one of the most highly prized of these tonic herbs. In particular, ashwagandha can relieve stress, which Ayurvedic healers have long recognized as a major cause of disease (see page 5).

Brahmi

Long before enlightened western physicians uttered the phrase "body/mind medicine," Ayurvedic healers knew that the underlying cause of many common problems—both physical and mental—is rooted in stress. As a result, many herbs that are used to treat a variety of ailments are also natural tranquilizers. Brahmi (also known as gotu kola) is a case in point. This herb, which has a mild tranquilizing effect, seems to work wonders on a number of different problems. Historically, brahmi has been the treatment of choice for problems related to mental function and nervous conditions. It is reputed to rejuvenate the brain and sharpen thinking. Brahmi is also a traditional treatment for skin disorders such as eczema and psoriasis, which we now know can be worsened by stress.

Gugul

In the West, where we like to place drugs in neat categories, gugul is described as an herb that can prevent heart disease because it reduces both high blood cholesterol and triglyceride levels. Ayurvedic practitioners feel that this approach is much too narrow. They view gugul as an herb that can strengthen the body in many different ways, and they fear that gugul's reputation as a lipid buster has overshadowed its other attributes. For example, gugul can enhance immune function, as is demonstrated by its ability to boost white blood cells. Ayurvedic practitioners would include gugul in formulas designed to strengthen and fortify many different body systems (see page 74).

Momordica Chirantia

Also known as bitter melon, this herb has traditionally been used by Ayurvedic healers to treat Type II, or adult-onset, diabetes. Numerous studies have shown that it can normalize elevated blood sugar levels. Indian researchers claim that it may boost the production or enhance the activity of insulin, the key hormone involved in the breakdown of sugar. There is exciting news about bitter melon as a potential treatment for AIDS and cancer. In test tube studies, bitter melon has stopped the replication of HIV, which causes AIDS. Bitter melon also stimulates the activity of disease-fighting immune cells. This effect suggests that bitter melon may help slow down the progress of AIDS and other diseases in humans. I recently learned that in San Francisco, there is a Bitter Melon Club organized by AIDS patients who are convinced that this herb, among other therapies, is helping to keep their disease in check. Bitter melon has also been shown to inhibit the growth of cancerous tumors in animals, and it also holds great promise as a cancer treatment. Fresh bitter melon is available from Asian grocery stores and is also sold in extract and capsules.

Picorhiza Kurroa

This herb is the traditional treatment for liver ailments and is also prescribed to support liver function. It is believed to protect the liver by inhibiting inflammatory processes, which can destroy liver cells. Although Ayurveda emphasizes using the whole plant, many herbs, including picorhiza kurroa, have been analyzed by researchers interested in developing drugs from individual compounds or in seeking scientific validity for this ancient system of medicine. Researchers have reported that picorhiza kurroa contains a substance called kutkin, which has a powerful protective effect on the liver. In one study involving patients with a parasitic infection, kutkin decreased the levels of harmful lipid peroxides (caused by free radicals) and increased the levels of superoxide dismutase (SOD), an important antioxidant, in the liver. This suggests that kutkin can help the liver to heal itself.

Shatawari

A member of the asparagus family, shatawari (which literally means "who possess 100 husbands") is a popular tonic reputed to enhance a woman's sexual vitality. This herb is used by women of all ages, from young adulthood through menopause, to normalize hormones. It is also prescribed as a treatment for diabetes for both men and women.

Triphala

Triphala, the combination of dried fruits from three different plants (amalaki, bibtaki, and haritaki), is the most widely used herbal preparation in Ayurvedic medicine. It can be taken alone or in combination with other herbs. Ayurvedic practitioners have dubbed triphala "good manager of the house" because it helps to harmonize the different bodily functions. In particular, triphala is reputed to normalize digestion, enhance nutrient absorption, and regulate metabolism. In one recent Indian study, triphala was successfully used to promote weight loss.

A Hot Tibetan Herb: Andrographis Paniculata

Rooted in the Ayurvedic tradition, Tibetan medicine is an intriguing blend of Indian, Chinese, and Greek medicine. Recently, there has been great interest in one particular Tibetan herb, andrographis paniculata, which is now available in natural food stores. For more than a decade, a cold remedy derived from andrographis has been used successfully in Nordic countries to reduce the severity and symptoms of the common cold. In fact, according to a double-blind study of 50 patients taking either andrographis or a placebo, more than half of those taking the andrographis extract reported that their symptoms were lighter than usual, and they recovered faster than those in the placebo group. In fact, after five days, 75 percent of the andrographis takers said that they were cured, while 40 percent of those in the placebo group were still battling cold symptoms.

Andrographis may also be of benefit to heart patients recovering from angioplasty, a common surgical procedure performed to clear plaque deposits from the arteries delivering blood to the heart, thereby improving blood flow. The major problem with angioplasty is that its effects are temporary, and the artery often becomes reclogged with plaque within several months after the procedure. This effect is called re-stenosis. Researchers at the Chinese Academy of Preventive Medicine discovered that administering andrographis to patients after angioplasty appeared to dramatically reduce the risk of re-stenosis by inhibiting the formation of new plaque.

What's even more exciting is that in test tube studies, a substance extracted from andrographis called andrographolide has been shown to inhibit human cancer cells in the breast, liver, and prostate. Unlike conventional chemotherapy drugs, which often have serious side effects, andrographolide is nontoxic. Researchers at the Rosell Park Cancer Institute in Syracuse, New York, are investigating the use of andrographolide as a treatment for prostate cancer, a type of cancer for which there is no cure and few effective treatments.

Look for andrographis in cold remedies and cardiovascular formulas.

Chinese Supplements

Similar to Ayurvedic medicine, traditional Chinese medicine does not focus on individual symptoms but views the human body as an entire system that needs careful management. At the core of Chinese medicine is the fundamental belief in yin and yang, or balance of energy within the body. According to traditional Chinese medicine, there are two opposing forces in the universe: yin, which is negative, and yang, which is positive. Everything (including all herbs) and everybody are characterized as either yin or yang. Yin types tend to be cool, calm, and quiet. Yang types are hot, stimulating, and energetic. A healthy body is one that strikes a balance between the opposing forces of yin and yang. Disease occurs when there is imbalance in the body, and it can be cured only when the balance is restored. The goal of Chinese medicine is to prevent those imbalances, thereby keeping patients healthy. In fact, in ancient China, wealthy families would pay doctors a retainer to keep them well. If a family member got sick, it was a sign that the doctor wasn't doing his job, and he didn't get paid.

Traditional Chinese healers rely on herbal medicine, exercise, acupuncture, and meditation. Modern Chinese physicians often incorporate traditional Chinese medicine into their philosophy and practice.

The first Chinese herbal dates back to 3494 B.C., when experts under the direction of Emperor Shen Nung documented the healing powers of more than 7,000 herbs. About 1,000 years ago, during the Song Dynasty, this information was updated, and information on 2,000 effective herbal combinations was published. Like Ayurvedic healers, Chinese healers believe in using tonics to maintain health and vitality.

Chinese medicine emphasizes using the whole plant rather than extracts of one or two active ingredients. Dr. James H. Zhou, Ph.D., co-founder of HerbaSway, a producer of standardized Chinese herbs, notes that many herbs with proven health benefits, such as ginkgo biloba, actually contain chemicals that if used alone can be toxic. However, when combined with other chemicals found in the plant, these "bad" chemicals are neutralized and may even be helpful. True Chinese healers do not use herbs individually, but combine them in formulas with other herbs.

Until very recently, Chinese herbs were available only from Chinese herb shops, usually known only to other Chinese healers. Even if you could locate one in your area, the array of roots and dried herbs would be totally bewildering to all but a few knowledgeable practitioners. Today, it is much easier to use Chinese herbs. In fact, there are several brands of Chinese herbal products available at natural food stores. Herbs may be sold individually or in combination with other herbs designed to treat specific symptoms. There have been a few distressing reports of herbs imported from China that were of poor quality or even contaminated. To ensure quality, look for standardized products that ensure purity and potency, preferably from well-established companies.

Here are some popular Chinese herbs that can be found at your natural food store. Some have already achieved Hot 100 status; the others are worth watching.

Astralagus

Astralagus (also called huang chi) is known as an adaptogen, an herb that helps restore balance in the body as well as strengthen bodily functions. Modern research has discovered that astralagus has a powerful effect on immune function. Chinese physicians prescribe it to cancer patients to boost immunity after chemotherapy or radiation. Astralagus is used in herbal formulas designed to restore energy and stamina.

Chinese Knotweed

This Chinese herb not only helps relieve colds and coughs but also lowers blood pressure by improving circulation throughout the body. This heart-healthy herb may also reduce the risk of blood clots, thereby helping to prevent heart attack and stroke. In addition, Chinese herbalists prescribe this herb to relieve back pain. Look for Chinese knotweed (*Polygonum cuspidatum*) in formulas designed to boost cardiovascular health and in cold formulas.

Fo-Ti

Also known as he-shou-wu, this herb is reputed to be a great rejuvenator. According to Chinese folklore, it can restore youthful vitality and fertility and can even help prevent hair from turning gray. Fo-ti is also a traditional treatment for gastrointestinal problems and diabetes.

Gian Jiang (Ginger)

Known by Westerners as ginger, gian jiang is a "hot" or yang herb that has been a traditional treatment for motion sickness, flu, and gastrointestinal disorders. Ginger is particularly good for upset stomach and cramps. Chinese healers recommend ginger tea to pregnant women who are suffering from nausea related to morning sickness. The warmth exerted by ginger is believed to help rid the body of cold symptoms and respiratory infections. Gingerol, a compound in ginger, is a powerful antioxidant.

Ginger is available in capsules and combination formulas.

Horny Goat Weed

This is the traditional Chinese herb for lowering blood pressure and treating male impotence. It contains several compounds, including the flavonoid quercetin, which can improve circulation of blood throughout the body. As I mentioned in the section "Supplements to Jump-Start Your Sex Life," poor circulation is a major cause of sexual problems in men. Look for horny goat weed in male potency herbal products as well as products for cardiovascular health.

Immature Bitter Orange

A member of the citrus family, this herb has been used to treat digestive problems, coughs, allergies, and inflammatory conditions. Today, you will find immature bitter orange included in herbal combinations to treat allergies and cold symptoms. It contains a potent antioxidant called nobelitin.

Kudzu

This Hot 100 herb is being marketed in the West as a treatment for alcohol abuse and hangovers. Used for thousands of years by Chinese healers, kudzu also contains pueratin, a compound that helps improve blood flow and strengthen the heart. Chinese researchers report that kudzu may be a useful treatment for glaucoma, a condition caused by high ocular pressure, which can lead to blindness.

Lo Han Kuo

Known by the botanical name cucurbitaceae fruit, this fruit has been dubbed the magic herb. Chinese healers recommend it for colds, coughs, digestive problems, and stress relief. Sold as an extract in the United States, this herb has a naturally sweet taste—250 times sweeter than sugar, but with no calories. It can be used as a sweetener in beverages.

Ma Huang

Ma huang is the traditional Chinese remedy for asthma, colds, and other respiratory ailments. In fact, the Western drugs ephedrine and pseudoephedrine, which are commonly found in over-the-counter cold preparations, are compounds derived from ma huang. Ma huang is a "hot" or yang herb. In fact, it speeds up metabolism and is used in the West in some herbal weight-loss formulas. Although ma huang has been used safely in China for 4,000 years, there have been reports of teens using it to get high. If taken in excess, ma huang can have an amphetamine-like effect, causing the heart to race and blood pressure to rise. This herb should definitely not be used by people with heart problems. Use ma huang with caution, and only when you need it.

Wu-Wei-Tzu

Known as schisandra in the West, this herb is believed to be an adaptogen that can fortify and strengthen the body, enhancing resistance to disease and stress. Schisandra is included in sports supplements designed to increase stamina and improve athletic performance. You will also find it in tonics to improve overall health and vitality.

Supplements from the Rainforest

When historians look back on the twentieth century, the important things that we neglected to do may far out-weigh what we actually did. One critical area in which we are dragging our heels is saving the world's precious rainforests, particularly in the southern hemisphere. Within the past 20 years, half of the rainforests have vanished, being cleared away or logged at a rate of 320 square miles daily. Tragically, these rainforests contain more than 200,000 species of plants, of which only a few thousand have yet been identified. Nevertheless, about 25 percent of our pharmaceutical drugs are derived from rainforest plants, including many of our most effective cancer treatments, such as drugs used to treat childhood leukemia, vincristisine and vinblastine, derived from the rosy periwinkle tree, which has increased the survival rate in children from 20 percent to 80 percent. Imagine how many powerful cures are still waiting to be discovered but may be destroyed before we can get to them! In addition, the rainforest produces as much as 20 percent of the world's oxygen—another precious resource that is vital to our very survival.

Fortunately, there is a growing appreciation of the rainforest, and the countries of the world are putting pressure on local governments to halt the destruction of this natural pharmacy. As a result, the destruction has slowed down. But if we are not vigilant, it will pick up again, and lives that could have been saved will be lost.

Although many of the rainforest herbs are treatments for serious diseases, some are wonderful remedies for everyday ailments. Here is a review of some interesting herbs from the rainforest that can be purchased at your local natural food stores and can certainly enhance the quality of life.

Abuta

Known throughout the Amazon as the midwife's herb, abuta has been traditionally used to treat menstrual cramps, PMS, threatened miscarriages, and complications of childbirth. Abuta is believed to normalize hormone levels in women as well as relieve pain. You can find abuta included in herbal formulas promoted as female tonics or designed to treat menstrual problems.

Cajueiro

Also known as cashew fruit, cajueiro is rich in vitamin C. It is used by Amazon healers to treat flu and colds, and also as an aphrodisiac. Cajueiro is included in tonics and in products designed to enhance energy and sexual function.

Chuchuhuasi

A natural anti-inflammatory agent, this herb is a traditional remedy for rheumatoid arthritis and osteoarthritis. The bark of this plant is being investigated as a potential arthritis drug by a leading pharmaceutical company. Chuchuhuasi is included in formulas designed to enhance sports performance (it reduces muscle pain after a hard workout) and to treat arthritis.

Hercampure

This rainforest herb is being promoted as a cure for high cholesterol and obesity. It is reputed to speed up metabolism and to help the body burn fat more efficiently, as well as to control appetite. Look for this herb in weight-loss formulas.

Jatoba Tree

The bark of the jatoba tree is a well-known treatment for *Candida albicans* or fungal infections as well as for respiratory and urinary tract infections. It is also reputed to be an herbal energizer that increases strength and stamina. Jatoba is sold as a tea, or in formulas designed to treat *Candida* infections and to protect the prostate.

Maca

Found in the Andes mountains, the root of this herb has been worshipped by the Incas for its aphrodisiac and energizing properties. Interestingly, maca is also used to relieve symptoms of stress, which can kill romance as well as rob us of our vitality. Today, maca is often included in sports supplements and other formulas designed to recharge and revitalize the body. In the United States, natural healers have used maca to treat chronic fatigue syndrome. Maca is rich in amino acids, calcium, zinc, and other vitamins.

Pata de Vaca

Native to Brazil, this herb is a natural treatment for diabetes. People who are diabetic often suffer from a condition called polyuria, or frequent urination. This herb reputedly normalizes the frequency of urination.

Taheebo

Also known as pau d'arco, this herb is used to treat *Candida albicans* or fungal infections. Lapachol, found in the bark of the pau d'arco tree, contains cancer-fighting compounds. It is also used as a treatment for parasitic infections. Look for taheebo in combination formulas designed to treat *Candida* infections.

8

Supplements for Sensational Skin

Within the past few years, there has been nothing less than a revolution in natural skin care products. Unlike their old-fashioned counterparts, which primarily cover up problems, these new cutting-edge products actually enhance the health and quality of skin. In fact, many contain the same vitamins, minerals, and antioxidants that can be taken internally but are redesigned to be absorbed right into the skin, where it is needed the most. Before I review some of the best of these new products, let me tell you a bit about skin and why taking care of it is so important.

Skin is the largest organ system in the body—it makes up about 10 percent of our body weight—and it is one of the hardest-working. Skin provides cover and protection for our internal organs, is essential for the production and storage of vitamin D, and works with the immune system to keep unwanted viruses, bacteria, and other pathogens out of the body. In addition, skin helps us to maintain our body temperature and to retain blood and other body fluids.

Unlike other organs in the body, skin is constantly exposed to the environment. As a result, it begins to show signs of wear and tear as we age. Skin consists of two layers: the outer layer, or epidermis, and the inner layer, or dermis. Underneath the skin lies a subcutaneous layer of fatty tissue that separates our skin from our muscles and bones. The dermis is made up mainly of collagen, the tissue that provides the scaffolding that supports the outer layer of cells that form the epidermis. Several factors cause skin to age; one of the primary reasons skin begins to look older in midlife is a dramatic decline in collagen production. As the underlying layer of collagen shrinks, the top layer of skin begins to sag and wrinkle.

As we age, we do not make new cells as quickly or as efficiently as when we were young. The epidermis contains mature cells that are ready to be shed, and new cells are underneath waiting to replace them. The older we get, however, the longer it takes for these new cells to replace the old cells, and it shows. That is why older skin that is not well cared for can look dull and drab.

As we get older, skin also becomes drier because we lose cells that help the skin retain moisture; in fact, skin loses about 30 percent of its water content. Young cells are plump and full; older cells are dry and shriveled up.

Most damage to skin, however, including so-called laugh lines, crows' feet, and wrinkles, is due to exposure to the ultraviolet (UV) rays produced by the sun, or photoaging.

Damage from UV light is cumulative. Years can pass before its damaging effects become apparent. Generally, by the time we reach our mid-30s, the long-term effects of UV exposure start to become visible in the form of fine lines, wrinkles, and telltale changes in skin tone and color. Even if you don't sunbathe, you are getting a heavy dose of UV rays as you go about your daily business, every time you step out of the house.

There are two types of UV rays: UVA and UVB. Both types stimulate the formation of free radicals on the skin, which can cause as much damage on the outside of the body as they do on the inside.

UVB rays are commonly referred to as the "burning rays" because they can turn skin red and cause pain and inflammation.

UVA rays do not usually cause perceptible reddening of the epidermis, the outer layer of skin. Rather, UVA rays inflict their damage by injuring the cells of the dermis and the subcutaneous layer of fat that are underneath the outer layer. This causes the kind of hidden damage that shows up years later as lines and wrinkles, and sometimes even as skin cancer.

Our body's natural antioxidant defense network deactivates some free radicals before they can inflict harm, but antioxidant levels decline as we age. To compound the problem, numerous studies have shown that even a small amount of UV light—not even enough to give a blush to the skin—causes a steep drop in antioxidant levels. In other words, every time you expose your face to the sun, your skin is being robbed of the antioxidants that protect it and keep it healthy and young-looking.

Exposure to UV rays is the primary cause of skin cancer. Some 1,000,000 new cases of skin cancer are diagnosed each year in the United States. Wearing a sunblock or sunscreen can help protect against UV damage, but keep in mind that most sunscreens do not completely block out UVA rays. Although they may protect against UVB, the burning rays, the nonburning UVA rays are still damaging your skin. If you are outdoors for prolonged periods of time during the peak burning hours, 10 A.M. to 3 P.M., it is wise to wear a hat and to stay in the shade as much as possible.

As you may know, sunscreens are rated by SPF, or sun protection factor. A sun protection factor of 15 means that if it normally takes a person 10 minutes to burn, with an SPF of 15, he or she can stay out in the sun 15 times longer before burning. You should wear a sunscreen with an SPF of at least 15. Before you apply any sunscreen—or for that matter, any skin care product—to a sensitive area such as your face, test it first on a small patch of skin on your upper arm. Cover the area with a bandage and leave it on for 24 hours. If there is no sign of irritation, you can use it on other parts of your body.

The best way to maintain youthful, healthy skin is to protect it against the sun. In addition, there are many new products that can also help age-proof your skin and restore some of the important elements that time and nature have taken away.

Aloe Vera Gel

One key way to maintain healthy skin is to replenish lost moisture. Drinking eight glasses of filtered water daily is one way to make sure that your body is well hydrated. Using a good moisturizer, such as aloe vera, can also help your skin hold onto moisture. Aloe contains natural moisturizers called mucopolysaccharides, which are similar to the moisturizing cells found in the dermis that help retain moisture. It can also soothe irritated skin and promote healing of minor burns and wounds.

Alpha and Beta Hydroxy Acids

Out with the old—in with the new. That is the principle behind alpha and beta hydroxy acid creams and gels. AHAs and BHAs can penetrate the surface of the skin and "unglue" old cells, stimulating new cell growth. Over time, consistent use of an AHA or BHA will make skin look younger and fresher, and reduce the appearance of fine lines and wrinkles. Numerous AHA and BHA products are sold in pharmacies and natural food stores. AHAs are naturally occurring substances that are found in fruit, juice, sugar, wine, and milk. The most commonly used AHAs are lactic acid (from sour milk) and glycolic acid (from sugar cane). BHAs contain salicylic acid. AHAs can also increase the number of complex sugar molecules in the skin called glycoaminoglycans (GAGs), which help skin retain moisture.

AHAs and BHAs come in different strengths. I do not recommend using a product that has more than a 10 percent concentration of AHAs or BHAs. If you have very sensitive skin, start out by using a product that contains less than 5 percent. Some of these products may sting momentarily when you use them. This is normal, but if you have undue irritation—that is, reddening of the skin that doesn't go away within a minute or two— discontinue use.

AHAs and BHAs can make skin very sensitive to UV light. Therefore, if you use them, you must use a sunscreen or a sunblock every day. If you won't wear a sunscreen or a sunblock, do not use these products.

Ascorbic Acid (Vitamin C)

When my friend the late Linus Pauling popularized vitamin C as the cure for the common cold in the 1970s, he had no idea that this vitamin would one day be promoted as the cure for the common wrinkle. How amused he would be to know that today, vitamin C is the hottest new antiaging cosmetic to come about in years! Studies

show that vitamin C skin products can make a real difference not only in the appearance of your skin but in its
health and quality.

Vitamin C skin products can do what was once considered impossible: stimulate the growth of new collagen.
Vitamin C is essential for the production of new collagen, but as we age, there is a decline in the amount of
available vitamin C in the skin. When taken orally, most
of the vitamin C is used systemically and does not get
to skin cells. Several studies show that high-potency
vitamin C creams (over 10 percent concentration of vitamin C) can increase the level of this important vitamin
in the skin. Animal studies conducted at Duke University Medical Center show that skin cells treated with
vitamin C actually become thicker, which is a sign of collagen regeneration. Applying vitamin C directly to the
skin will help restore skin tone, plump up wrinkles, and
fill in small lines, giving skin a more youthful look. Topically applied vitamin C improves blood supply to the
skin, giving the skin a more youthful glow.

Vitamin C can minimize fine lines, reduce light wrinkles, and improve skin color and tone, which will result
in a more taut, less flabby look.

In addition, vitamin C has been shown to protect skin
from damage inflicted by UV light and to reduce some of
the inflammation caused by UV exposure. In fact, studies
have shown that topically applied vitamin C can prevent
one of the most dangerous effects of UV exposure: the
suppression of the immune system. This means that vitamin C not only has a cosmetic effect but offers serious
protection against further damage to the skin.

Vitamin C should be used only in specially formulated
products designed specifically for external use. Otherwise,
it will not be absorbed by the skin. Do not rub vitamin C

from a pill or capsule directly onto the skin; it could be very irritating, not to mention totally ineffective. Vitamin C is available as a liquid serum or a cream. Since potent vitamin C serums and creams may cause discomfort if they get into the eyes, weaker versions of the serum and cream are designed to be used around the delicate eye area.

The serums are stronger than the creams and are therefore more effective. However, people with very sensitive skin may find them to be too irritating and may prefer to use a cream.

If you have age-related damage near your eyes, you should use a milder vitamin C cream or gel designed for use around the eyes in addition to the stronger gel or cream you use on the rest of your skin.

Chamomile

Proper cleansing is essential for glowing, healthy skin. Too often, however, people make the mistake of over-cleansing: they use harsh detergent-like or abrasive products that not only are irritating but strip the skin of important oils. Chamomile is a wonderful gentle cleanser that is usually tolerated by even the most sensitive skin. Look for products that list chamomile as a primary ingredient, such as CamuCare Chamomile Cleansing Therapy or Basis Soap, which are sold in pharmacies or health food stores.

Emu Oil

Long used by Aboriginal healers in Australia to treat wounds and burns, emu oil (from the emu bird) is now being promoted as a moisturizer for the skin that can also protect against sun damage. In addition, emu oil is reputed to reduce fine lines and wrinkles. Look for it in cosmetics and skin care products.

Essential Fatty Acids

Show me someone who is on an extremely low-fat diet, and I will show you someone who has dry skin and dull, lifeless hair. Some fat in your diet is absolutely essential for healthy, glowing skin. In particular, essential fatty acids, such as gamma linoleic acid, help the skin retain its elasticity and seal in moisture. Several of the supplements I have already reviewed (flaxseed oil, conjugated linoleic acid, omega-3 fatty acids, evening primrose oil) are essential fatty acids. However, if you have dry skin, it is also important to use an external moisturizer with essential fatty acids for best results. Read the product labels to see if the moisturizers contain essential fatty acids. I don't recommend opening up capsules of essential fatty acids that are meant to be taken orally. These products not only are too greasy to be pleasant to use but may not be as well absorbed as a product specifically designed for external use. Products also containing liposomes and hyaluronic acid are good choices because they help to deliver moisture more effectively to the deep cells within the skin.

Green Tea Extract

Recently, numerous studies have confirmed that compounds in green tea called polyphenols can protect against cancer. In fact, when applied to the skin of animals, green tea polyphenols have been shown to prevent skin tumors from forming after exposure to known carcinogens and excessive sunlight. Skin creams containing green tea poly-phenols are now being sold at natural food stores. In addition to fighting cancer, green tea skin care products are very soothing and are especially good for sensitive or irritated skin. Several people have told me that these green tea products can help reduce minor irritation caused by some of the antiaging skin care products (such as AHAs, BHAs, retinol, and vitamin C cream) that work below the top layers of skin.

Kinetin

Kinetin, a growth hormone extracted from plants, is being used in skin creams and gels. In test tube studies, kinetin has been shown to extend the life of human skin fibroblasts, which are believed to be instrumental in skin aging. Fibroblasts produce collagen and elastin, which are important for maintaining the texture and tone of skin. Skin products containing kinetin may also include vitamins and antioxidants.

Oxygen Cream

Energy is necessary for the production of new cells and the repair of old cells. Oxygen, which is essential for the production of energy, is delivered to cells via the blood, which travels through tiny capillaries. As we age, the capillary network weakens and becomes less efficient. As a result, the blood supply to many different organ systems, especially the skin, is diminished. The net effect is that our skin begins to look old and tired. The cure? Breathe new life into worn-out skin with face creams that deliver oxygen directly into skin cells.

Oxygen skin products contain hydrogen peroxide, which is broken down into oxygen when it comes in contact with skin. Studies show that after even one application of hydrogen peroxide, skin levels of oxygen rise dramatically. Oxygen facials, in which a jet of pure oxygen is actually blown on the face, are now being offered in cutting-edge salons across the country.

Critics of oxygen creams and treatments contend that they have little effect on the quality of skin, but people who use these products keep coming back for more. All I can say is that if you're interested, you should try it, and see if it helps. (Although oxygen is critical for energy production, as I mentioned earlier, it also promotes the formation of free radicals. Therefore, oxygen skin products often contain antioxidants to "mop up" any potentially troublesome free radicals. In my opinion, if you breathe, you should be taking antioxidants!)

Proanthocyanidins (PCOs) Cream and Gel

Proanthocyanidins (PCOs), derived from pine trees grown in France that are rich in antioxidants, are now available for use on the skin. Several brands of skin creams and gels (such as DERMA E) include PCOs, usually in combination with other antioxidants such as vitamin E.

PCOs help maintain healthy, beautiful skin in several important ways. First, the flavonoids in PCOs help to strengthen capillaries, the tiny blood vessels that deliver blood and nutrients to tissues and cells in your body, including those in the skin. As we age, these tiny capillaries begin to break down, resulting in diminished blood flow. Fortifying these tiny blood vessels will improve circulation throughout the body, including the skin.

As I mentioned earlier, skin aging is primarily caused by free radical attack, which breaks down collagen, the underlying protein that supports the outer layers of skin. As we age, skin begins to sag and wrinkle because of the loss of collagen fibers. Studies have shown that PCOs can help protect collagen against free radical attack and even stimulate collagen repair. In one study, collagen fibers were soaked in water for 24 hours with a weight attached to them so that they would become weakened and stretched, to mimic the effect of adding decades of wear and tear to the skin. However, when PCOs were added to the water, the fibers actually shortened and became stronger, suggesting that PCOs would rejuvenate skin.

Because they are rich in antioxidants, PCOs also provide added protection against damaging UV rays. In one study performed in Finland, human skin cells were exposed to UV radiation. Without any protection, after prolonged exposure, about 50 percent of the skin cells died. However, when PCOs were added to the cells, 85 percent of them survived the UV radiation. In particular, PCOs can protect against dangerous UVB rays, which are responsible for sunburn and for damage to the epidermis, the outer layer of skin.

PCOs enhance the action of vitamin C, another essential vitamin for youthful, glowing skin. PCOs are sold in capsules to be taken orally, but using the cream or gel is a more efficient way to deliver PCOs directly to the skin.

Retinol Cream

Vitamin A has long been known as the vitamin for beautiful skin. The first vitamin A cream was tretinoin, better known as Retin-A, which was originally used as an acne treatment, but dermatologists who treated adults with Retin-A noticed that it also improved fine lines and wrinkles. More recently, another type of vitamin A cream—retinoic acid, marketed as Renova—became the first FDA-approved prescription wrinkle cream. Although these prescription products work very well, the downside is that they can be irritating and can cause skin to redden and peel.

Now, a weaker cousin of retinoic acid, retinol, is being sold over the counter. Like Retin-A and Renova, retinol can help to reduce fine lines and wrinkles and reduce age-associated skin discolorations without the troublesome side effects. Like AHAs, retinol sloughs off old cells and stimulates the formation of new cells. Retinol is unique in that it can do something more than these other products do: it can "reprogram" the new cells to act more like cells on young skin. The new cells not only look younger but will retain moisture the way that younger skin cells do. In one study conducted by Neutrogena, which has recently introduced Neutrogena Healthy Skin Anti-Wrinkle Cream (a retinol product), people who used retinol for 12 weeks showed a real improvement in over-all skin texture and reduction of fine wrinkles, especially around the eyes. The before-and-after photographs are quite impressive. The best news is that since retinol is not as strong as the prescription vitamin A products, it is not nearly as irritating, although it may cause minor redness and some flaking in the sensitive skin of some people. Several retinol skin products are sold in pharmacies and natural food stores. Several of them include vitamin C, vitamin E, or other antioxidants.

Tea Tree Oil

There is nothing more unsightly than chipped, peeling, or discolored nails caused by a fungal infection. Nail fungus is particularly persistent and difficult to treat. Tea tree oil is a time-honored remedy for fungal infections that is widely used in the tropics. When applied directly to the nail, tea tree can help speed recovery, especially when used in conjunction with other treatments, such as surgical debridement, removal of the infected tissue. Once the infection is gone, tea tree oil can also help prevent its recurrence.

Tea tree oil is also used in antidandruff shampoos. Recently, studies have shown that yeast infections may aggravate psoriasis and eczema, two skin conditions that can result in a dry, flaky scalp. If you are prone to yeast infections, tea tree oil shampoo may help keep your scalp clear.

Tocopherol (Vitamin E)

When the antiaging properties of vitamin E became widely known in the 1980s, people would cut open vitamin E capsules and rub the oil directly on their skin to prevent wrinkles. (I don't recommend this: not only is vitamin E oil greasy, but it can be very irritating to some people.) Cosmetic manufacturers got wind of this trend and put a small amount of vitamin E in their products. Unfortunately, in many cases, they didn't put in enough vitamin E to make a real difference. Now some new high-potency vitamin E creams are available that are non-greasy and are reportedly highly effective antiaging agents, especially for sensitive areas of the face. In one recent study, 20 women, aged 42 to 64, used a vitamin E cream over one wrinkled eyelid and a placebo cream over the other. Within four weeks, half of the women showed a greater decrease in the size and roughness of the wrinkled area treated with vitamin E than in the side treated with the placebo. Vitamin E has also been used to help fade scars and reduce stretch marks.

Vitamin K Cream

Vitamin K cream is used to help fade spider veins, broken capillaries, and bruises and to speed healing in sun-damaged skin. It is sometimes used following cosmetic surgical procedures such as laser resurfacing, to prevent postoperative scarring. Vitamin K cream is somewhat expensive, and the reviews are mixed. Some people swear by it; others say it doesn't work for them.

9

Get Smarter with Supplements

A friend who had recently turned 50 and had just started a new job found much to his chagrin that he was having difficulty remembering the names of his new co-workers. Not only that, but he felt that he wasn't quite as sharp as he used to be. "Tell me what to take, and I'll take it!" he begged.

I compiled a list of supplements that I knew would help, and at the same time, I reassured him that his experience was typical. As people age they are likely to experience some change in mental function, but these changes are fairly minor. The decline in short-term memory is very common, and although forgetting the names of new acquaintances or phone numbers may be annoying, it is not serious. I also stressed that with proper intervention, these problems need never become serious. With the exception of the minority of older people who develop a serious brain disorder such as Alzheimer's disease, most of us can maintain good brain function for our entire lives.

But staying sharp entails more than just swallowing a few pills. Your mental state is often very much a reflection of your physical state. If you are active, healthy, and vigorous, chances are you will be able to function well, mentally and physically. In fact, physical problems are often the underlying cause of many supposedly mental problems. For example, atherosclerosis, which interferes with the flow of blood to the brain, can result in a noticeable decline in mental capacity. High blood pressure can have a similar effect.

I cannot overemphasize the role of diet in brain function. Your brain requires constant nourishment to fuel its many activities. At any age, if you eat erratically or if you do not get enough nutrients, your brain cells will not have the energy to perform well. Numerous studies have shown that when students skip breakfast, they fare poorly in school. Obviously, it is very difficult to concentrate or to feel energetic when you are hungry.

Sometimes you may be "hungry" for a specific nutrient and not realize it. For example, many people over the age of 60 are deficient in vitamin B_{12}. This deficiency may be responsible for certain neurologic symptoms ranging from weakness to lack of balance, mood changes, disorientation, and memory loss. In fact, according to a study performed in the Netherlands, healthy people with lower blood levels of vitamin B_{12} don't perform as well on mental tests as people with higher levels. And it's not just older people in whom nutrient deficiencies can affect mental function; younger people are also vulnerable. For example, iron deficiency has been shown to lower the test scores of college students. Students at Penn State who were found to be deficient in iron took iron supplements for three months and significantly increased their test scores.

A lack of physical activity can also cause the brain to stagnate. Physical inactivity is accompanied by electrical and chemical changes in the brain that lead to decreased levels of two neurotransmitters, dopamine and noradrenaline, which are essential for alertness. Exercise reverses that decrease by increasing the availability of oxygen to the brain. Exercise strengthens the pumping action of the heart, which improves circulation. In addition to increasing oxygen stores, exercise creates a natural high. It stimulates the release of endorphins, neurochemicals that actually have an opiate-like effect on the brain. People who exercise think more clearly, feel more alert and energetic, and have a markedly increased sense of well-being.

Exercise also helps relieve stress, which can have a detrimental effect on brain function. Numerous studies have shown that prolonged stress can accelerate brain aging and even damage areas of the brain involved in learning and memory. Researchers at McGill University in Montreal monitored the concentration of the blood levels of stress hormones in 130 healthy volunteers, from 55 to 87 years old, over a five-year period. The researchers discovered that high blood levels of stress hormones correlated with subtle memory and attention problems. High levels of stress hormones have even been suggested as a possible cause of Alzheimer's disease.

Clearly, maintaining your mental acuity goes hand in hand with maintaining a healthy lifestyle. Here are some supplements that will help you do both.

Antioxidants Protect Your Brain

Your brain is composed of more than 50 percent fatty tissue, which makes it especially vulnerable to attack by free radicals, unstable oxygen molecules that are normal byproducts of the cells' use of oxygen. In fact, the destruction of brain cells by free radicals is believed to be a causative factor in many different diseases of the brain, including Alzheimer's and Parkinson's. When we are young, our bodies have a strong network of antioxidants that can ward off destructive free radicals, but as we age, our levels of naturally produced antioxidants decline. That is why it is important to take supplemental antioxidants. Antioxidants are sold separately or in combination formulas. These are some of the best antioxidants for your brain.

Grapeseed Extract

Rich in proanthocyanidins, which are similar to flavonoids, grapeseed extract can help protect fat cells from troublesome free radicals. It also helps to prevent heart disease by protecting collagen, which is essential for healthy arteries. Take up to two tablets daily.

Vitamin E

For years, I have been impressed by the fact that older people who take vitamin E seem to be more on the ball than those who don't. Now I know why. Vitamin E, a potent antioxidant, has a powerful effect on the brain. In one study, patients with early Alzheimer's disease of moderate severity were given either a prescription drug (selegine), vitamin E (2000 IU), a combination of both, or a placebo for two years. After evaluating the patients at the end of the study, the researchers concluded that vitamin E alone, even better than the prescription drugs, could slow down the progress of Alzheimer's disease. Not only does vitamin E protect against free radicals, but it also helps ward off heart disease, which can accelerate the destruction of brain cells.

In another fascinating study, rats were given the human equivalent of 400 IU of vitamin E daily. Researchers reported that after the rats ingested vitamin E, a protein found in the brains of the rats (and humans as well) did not suffer the type of oxidative "wear and tear" that would ordinarily have occurred in association with brain aging. They concluded that vitamin E may help keep an "old" brain young! Take 400 IU of dry vitamin E daily.

Lipoic Acid

Lipoic acid is known as the universal antioxidant because it can enhance the activity of other antioxidants in the body. It is also unique because it is neither fat-soluble nor water-soluble, which means it can get into every part of every cell. While other antioxidants are highly specialized and are effective against only one or two different free radicals, lipoic acid is able to quench (or defuse) many different types of free radicals. It is also able to pass through the blood-brain barrier, enabling it to help repair injured brain cells. In fact, animal studies show that lipoic acid can totally reverse the negative effects to the brain caused by a stroke, the temporary deprivation of blood and oxygen that can cause severe memory loss and confusion. This makes sense—much of the damage inflicted by a stroke is actually caused by the proliferation of free radicals. I predict that lipoic acid will soon become known as the key antioxidant for brain health. Take up to 100 mg. of lipoic acid daily.

NADH

Also known as coenzyme 1, NADH is an antioxidant that shows promise as a tonic for the brain. Interestingly, Alzheimer's patients have NADH levels 25 to 50 percent lower than in people of the same age who remain free of Alzheimer's. In one study, Alzheimer's patients given 10 mg. of NADH daily showed a noticeable improvement in cognitive function and memory. Take up to two 5-mg. tablets daily on an empty stomach.

B Stands for "Brain"

As I mentioned earlier, numerous studies have shown that low levels of B vitamins can cause subtle changes in brain function among older people that could contribute to memory loss and even depression. Folic acid, in particular, may prevent memory loss by helping to maintain normal levels of homocysteine, an amino acid found in the body. High levels of homocysteine are believed to increase the risk of heart disease. In addition, a recent study performed by the Agriculture Research Service of the U.S. Department of Agriculture found a strong correlation between high blood levels of homocysteine and the loss of memory and ability to learn that often accompanies depression in the elderly.

Take one 50-mg. vitamin B complex capsule or tablet daily with 400 mcg. folic acid, one 500-mg. vitamin B_1 or thiamine capsule daily, and one 1000-mcg. vitamin B_{12} tablet in sublingual form (dissolved under the tongue).

Choline

The cells of the brain "talk" to each other by releasing chemicals called neurotransmitters, of which one of the most important is acetylcholine. As we age, we experience a decline in neurotransmitters by as much as 70 percent, which may also be a factor in brain aging. Researchers suspect that choline supplements can help to retard the effects of normal aging on the brain from midlife on.

Choline is utilized by the brain to make acetylcholine, which is involved in memory function, and it may also keep nerve cell membranes, including the synapses (the communication points between brain cells) intact, which enables brain cells to "talk" to each other and share information.

As we age, we begin to produce less acetylcholine, or the acetylcholine that we do produce is less efficient, which may be why many older people become forgetful. The utilization of choline in the body depends on several other nutrients, principally vitamin B_{12}, folic acid, and the amino acid L-carnitine.

Choline may be sold under the name of phosphatidylcholine or phosphatidylinositol. Use whichever is easier for you to find. Take between 1000 and 3000 mg. daily.

L-Carnitine

The body uses L-carnitine to produce the enzyme acetyl-L-carnitine transferase, which boosts choline metabolism and releases acetylcholine in the brain. Good food sources of L-carnitine include eggs, soybeans, cabbage, peanuts, and cauliflower. Take up to 3 mg. of L-carnitine daily.

DHA

There's a reason why fish is known as brain food. It is a rich source of docosahexaenoic acid (DHA), a fatty acid that is found in high concentration in the gray matter of the brain. DHA is instrumental in the function of brain cell membranes, which are important for the transmission of brain signals. Over the past century, there has been a steady decline in DHA consumption. Take three 250-mg. capsules daily.

DMAE

Dimethylaminoethanol (DMAE), which is produced in the body, is another supplement that can boost acetylcholine, thereby enhancing memory and mental function. Although it can be taken alone, DMAE is often used in formulas designed to improve cognitive function. DMAE is one of the few substances that can cross the blood-brain barrier and get right to the brain cells where it is needed. Recently, DMAE has been shown to be effective for children with attention deficit disorder (ADD) and is being promoted as a natural alternative to Ritalin, the drug often prescribed for this problem. Take one to two tablets daily. I take a combination formula of DMAE, ginkgo biloba, phosphatidylserine, inositol, and choline daily.

Ginkgo Biloba

The ginkgo tree, which dates back to before the Ice Age, is a rich source of bioflavonoids (potent antioxidants) and other components that have many medicinal properties. In animal studies, ginkgo has been shown to increase the levels of dopamine, a chemical found in the brain that improves the body's ability to transmit information.

Ginkgo also appears to have a "brain-boosting" effect in humans. Ginkgo biloba has been studied as a treatment for inadequate blood flow to the brain, and the results are extremely promising. In one recent French study, a group of 60- to 80-year-olds who had slight problems with mental function were given ginkgo biloba supplements or a placebo. One hour later they took a battery of tests to determine their speed of information processing. After treatment with ginkgo biloba, the patients' scores improved so dramatically that they were close to the scores of young, healthy people.

Take up to three 60-mg. standardized capsules daily.

Gotu Kola

Also known as brahmi, this herb has been used in India and China for thousands of years. Recent studies show that gotu kola has a positive effect on the circulatory system by strengthening the veins and capillaries, thereby improving the flow of blood throughout the body, including the brain. Look for gotu kola in combination formulas designed to boost brain power.

Huperzine A and B

Derived from club moss tea, these compounds have been found to be potent natural memory enhancers. Researchers at the Shanghai Institute of Materia Medica reported that huperzine A and huperzine B can help improve learning, memory retrieval, and memory retention. Look for huperzine A and B (or club moss tea) in formulas designed to enhance mental function.

Magnesium

This mineral can prevent many of the problems that lead to impaired mental function, such as atherosclerosis and high blood pressure. Magnesium is also critical for nerve cell regulation and plays a role in controlling the activity of neurons. Magnesium deficiency has been associated with ADD in children and adults. Most Americans do not get enough magnesium, and magnesium intake is actually on the decline. Protect yourself against magnesium deficiency by taking 250 to 500 mg. daily.

Pregnenolone

Researchers have found that estrogen, testosterone, and DHEA, the hormones associated with reproductive activity, are also neurotransmitters and play a major role in maintaining mood and mental function. In fact, the decline in these hormones is in part responsible for some of the age-related changes that occur in brain function.

A new natural hormone, pregnenolone, is now being sold over the counter and is reputed to be the most potent memory-enhancing agent to date. In recent animal studies, researchers were very excited because only a few molecules of this hormone vastly improved the memory of mice—a strong indication that it would also work well in humans. In reality, pregnenolone already has a pretty good track record in humans. In the 1940s, pregnenolone was shown to enhance learning skills, elevate mood, and improve the performance of factory workers and airline pilots. At the time, pregnenolone was primarily being developed as a treatment for arthritis, and once cortisone was discovered, research on pregnenolone was discontinued. Lately, however, researchers have become interested in pregnenolone as an antiaging therapy. Pregnenolone is believed to be safe, and there are no known side effects. Take up to 50 mg. of pregnenolone daily.

Phosphatidylserine

I noted earlier that the brain contains a large amount of fatty tissue, or phospholipids, which makes it especially vulnerable to free radical attack. Restoring phospholipids can help boost brain function. Phospholipids not only hold the cells together but control the entrance and exit of substances in and out of the cells. They are also involved in communication among cells, which is a function of vital importance in the brain.

Phosphatidylserine is one of the most abundant phospholipids in the brain. Its primary role is to help relay chemical messages from brain cell to brain cell. Studies have shown that phosphatidylserine supplements can have a significantly positive effect on brain function. In one recent study, 149 healthy men and women, 50 to 70 years of age, were all diagnosed with normal age-associated memory impairment, the kind of forgetfulness we all experience as we grow older. Participants were given 100 mg. of phosphatidylserine (PS) daily for 12 weeks or a placebo. Those taking the PS noted significant improvements in their ability to do normal tasks, such as recall telephone numbers and names and faces. Those who took the placebo showed virtually no change.

Begin with a dose of 200 mg. of PS daily. After four weeks, cut down to 100 mg. daily.

Selected Bibliography

Abraham, G. E., et al. "Management of Fibromyalgia: Rationale for the Use of Magnesium and Malic Acid." *Journal of Nutri. Med.*, vol. 3 (1992): 49–50.

Adam, M. "What Effect Does a Protein Hydrolysate Preparation Have? Therapy for Osteoarthritis," *Therpiewoche* 39 (1989): 3153–57.

Altura, B., et al. "Magnesium: Growing in Clinical Importance." *Patient Care* (January 15, 1994): 130–50.

Anderson, R. A. "Chromium, Glucose Tolerance and Diabetes." *Biological Trace Element Research* 32 (1992): 19–24.

Baggio, E. R., et al. "Italian Multicenter Study on the Safety and Efficacy of Coenzyme Q10 as an Adjunctive Therapy in Heart Failure (interim analysis)." *Clinical Investigator* 71:S (1993): 145–49.

Barnes, S., et al. "Soybeans Inhibit Mammary Tumors in Models of Breast Cancer." *Mutagens and Carcinogens in Diet* (1990): 239–53.

Barrett-Connor, E., et al. "A Perspective Study of Dehydro-epiandrosterone Sulfate, Mortality and Cardiovascular Disease." *New England Journal of Medicine* 315, vol. 24 (April 11, 1986): 1519–24.

Batieha, A. M., et al. "Serum Micronutrients and the Subsequent Risk of Cervical Cancer in a Population-Based Nested

Case-Control Study." *Cancer Epidemiology, Biomarkers and Prevention* 2 (July/August 1993): 335–39.

Boman, G., et al. "Oral Acetylcysteine Reduces Exacerbation Rates in Chronic Bronchitis." *European Journal of Respiratory Diseases* 64 (1983): 405–15.

Braeckman, J. "The Extract of Serenoa Repens in the Treatment of Benign Prostatic Hyperplasis: A Multicenter Open Study." *Current Therapy Research* 55 (1994): 776–85.

Cangiano, C., et al. "Eating Behavior and Adherence to Dietary Prescriptions in Obese Subjects Treated with 5-Hydroxytryptophan." *American Journal of Clinical Nutrition* 56 (1992): 863–68.

Castleman, M. "Red Pepper Is Hot." *Medical Selfcare* (September–October 1989).

Champlault, G., et al. "A Double Blind Trial of an Extract of the Plant Serenoa Repens in Benign Prostatic Hyperplasia." *British Journal of Clinical Pharmacology* 18 (1984): 461–62.

Chandra, R. K. "Graying of the Immune System: Can Nutrient Supplements Improve Immunity in the Elderly?" *Journal of the American Medical Association* 277, no. 17 (May 7, 1997): 1398–99.

"Chronic Stress Is Directly Linked to Premature Aging of the Brain." *National Institute on Aging, Research Bulletin* (October 1991).

Cichoke, A. "Maitake: The King of Mushrooms." *Townsend Letter for Doctors* 130 (May 1994): 432–33.

———. "Probiotics Balance Digestion and Improve Overall Health." *Nutrition Science News*, vol. 2, no. 8 (August 1997): 380.

Clark, L. C., et al. "Effects of Selenium Supplementation for Cancer Prevention in Patients with Carcinoma of the Skin." *Journal of the American Medical Association* 276, vol. 24 (December 25, 1997): 1957–63.

Crimi, A., et al. "Extract of Serenoa Repens for the Treatment of the Functional Disturbances of Prostate Hypertrophy." *Med. Praxis* 4 (1983) 47–51.

Crook, T. H., et al. "Effects of Phosphatidylserine in Age-Associated Memory Impairment." *Neurology* 41 (1991): 644–49.

Di Luzio, N. R. "Immunopharmacology of Glucan: A Broad Spectrum Enhancer of Host Defense Mechanisms." *Trends in Pharmacological Sciences* 4 (1983): 344–47.

Ditre, M. Cherie, et al. "Effects of a-Hydroxy Acids on Photoaged Skin: A Pilot Clinical, Histologic and Ultrasound Study." *Journal of the American Academy of Dermatology* 34 (2) Part 1 (February): 187–95.

Earnest, C. P. "The Effect of Creatine Monohydrate Ingestion on Anaerobic Power Indices, Muscular Strength and Body Composition." *Acta Physiol. Scand.* 153 (1995): 207–9.

"Flax Facts." *Journal of the National Cancer Institute* 83, no. 15 (September 7, 1991): 1050–52.

Flodin, N. W., et al. "The Metabolic Roles, Pharmacology and Toxicity of Lysine." *American Journal of Clinical Nutrition*, vol. 16, no. 1 (1997): 7–21.

Flood, J. F., et al. "Memory Enhancing Effects in Male Mice of Pregnenolone and Steroids Metabolism Derived from It." *Proc. Nat. Acad. Sci. USA* 89 (1992): 1567–71.

Fotsis, T., et al. "Genistein, a Dietary Derived Inhibitor of In Vitro Angiogenesis." *Proc. Nat. Acad. Sci.* 90 (April 1993): 2690–94.

Frankel, P., et al. "Beyond Antioxidants: Methylation, Homocysteine and Nutrition." *The Research Corner* (1996).

Gao, Y. T., et al. "Reduced Risk of Esophageal Cancer Associated with Green Tea Consumption." *Journal of the National Cancer Institute* 86, no. 11 (June 1, 1994): 855–58.

Gibson, R. G., et al. "Perna Canaliculus in the Treatment of Arthritis." *The Practitioner* 224 (1980): 995–99.

Giovannucci, E., et al. "Intake of Carotenoids and Retinol in Relation to Risk of Prostate Cancer." *Journal of the National Cancer Institute* 87 (1995): 1767–76.

Hata, Y., et al. "Effects of Fructooligosaccharides (Neosugar) on Hyperlipidima." *Geriatric Medicine* 21 (1982): 156.

Herve, A., et al. "Effect of Two Doses of Ginkgo Biloba Extract (EGB 761) on the Dual-Coding Test in Elderly Subjects." *Clinical Therapeutics* 15, no. 3 (1993): 549–58.

Hierholzer, J. C., et al. "In Vitro Effects of Monolaurin Compounds on Enveloped RNA and DNA Viruses." *Journal of Food Safety* 4 (1982).

Jang, M., et al. "Chemoprotective Activity of Resveratrol, a Natural Product Derived from Grapes." *Science,* vol. 275 (January 10, 1997): 218–20.

Joosten, E., et al. "Metabolic Evidence That Deficiencies of Vitamin B-12 (Cobalamin), Folate and Vitamin B-6 Occur Commonly in Older People." *American Journal of Clinical Nutrition* 58 (1993): 468–76.

Julius, M., et al. "Glutathione and Morbidity in a Community-Based Sample of Elderly." *Journal of Clinical Epidemiology* 47, no. 9 (1994): 1021–26.

Kahn, R. S., et al. "L-5 Hydroxytryptophan in the Treatment of Anxiety Disorders." *Journal of Affective Disorders* 8 (1985): 197–200.

Kamikawa, T., et al. "Effects of Coenzyme Q10 on Exercise Tolerance in Chronic Stable Angina Pectoris." *American Journal of Cardiology* 56 (1985): 247–51.

Kang, S., et al. "The Cosmetic Beautifying Effect of Retinol (Vitamin A)." *Society for Investigative Dermatology* 105 (1995): 556.

Kanter, M. M., et al. "Antioxidants, Carnitine and Choline as Putative Erogenic Aids." *International Journal of Sports Nutrition* 5 (1995): S120–S131.

Kato, M., et al. "Induction of Gene Expression for Immunomodulating Cytokines in Peripheral Blood Mononuclear Cells in Response to Orally Administered PSK, an Immunomodulating Protein-Bound Polysaccharide." *Cancer Immunol. Immunother.* 40 (1995): 152–56.

Kleijnin, J., et al. "Ginkgo Biloba." *The Lancet* 340 (1992): 1136–39.

Kreider, R. B. "Effects of Ingesting Supplements Designed to Promote Lean Tissue Accretion on Body Composition

During Resistance Training." *International Journal of Sports Nutrition* 6: 234–46.

Lee, J. R. "Osteoporosis Reversal: The Role of Progesterone." *International Clinical Nutrition Review* 10 (1990): 384–91.

Loike, J. D., et al. "Extracellular Creatine Regulates Creatine Transport in Rat and Human Muscle Cells." *Proc. Nat. Acad. Sci. USA* 85 (February 1988): 807–11.

Messina, M., et al. "Soy Intake and Cancer Risk: A Review of the In Vitro and In Vivo Data." *Nutrition and Cancer* 21, no. 2 (1994).

Meydani, S. N., "Vitamin E." *The Lancet* 435 (January 21, 1995): 170–75.

Meydani, S. N., et al. "Vitamin E Supplementation and In Vivo Immune Response in Healthy Elderly Subjects: A Randomized Controlled Trial." *Journal of the American Medical Association* 227, no. 17 (May 7, 1997): 1380–85.

Michnovicz, J. J., et al. "Altered Estrogen Metabolism and Excretion in Humans Following Consumption of Indole-3 Carbinol." *Nutrition and Cancer* 16 (1991): 56–66.

Morales, A. J., et al. "Effect of Replacement Dose of DHEA in Men and Women of Advancing Age." *Journal of Clinical Endocrinology Metabolism* (1994): 1360–67.

Nagabhushan, M., et al. "Curcumin As an Inhibitor of Cancer." *Journal of the American College of Nutrition* 11 (1992): 192.

Nissen, S., et al. "Effect of Leucine B-Hydroxy-B-Methylbutyrate on Muscle Metabolism During Resistance Training." *Journal of Applied Physiology*, vol. 81, no. 5 (1996): 2095–2104.

Packer, L., et al. "Alpha-lipoic Acid As a Biological Agent." *Free Radical Biological Medicine* 19 (August 1995): 227–50.

Parry-Billings, M., et al. "A Communication Link Between Skeletal Muscle, Brain and Cells of the Immune System." *International Journal of Sports Medicine* 11 (1990): S122–S128.

Pederson, R., et al. "Long Term Effects of Vanadyl Treatment on Streptozotocin-Induced Diabetes in Rats." *Diabetes* 38 (1989): 1390–95.

Pierpaoli, W., et al. *The Melatonin Miracle.* New York: Simon & Schuster, 1995.

Pincus, G., et al. "Effects of Administered Pregnenolone on Fatiguing Psychomotor Performance." *Aviation Medicine* (April 1944): 98–135.

Pinnell, S., et al. "Induction of Collagen Synthesis by Ascorbic Acid: A Possible Mechanism." *Archives of Dermatology* (1987): 1684–86.

———. "Regulation of Collagen Biosynthesis by Ascorbic Acid: A Review." *Yale Journal of Biological Medicine* 58 (1985): 553–59.

Platt, D., et al. "Modulation of the Lung Colonization of B12-F1 Melanoma Cells by Citrus Pectin." *Journal of the National Cancer Institute* 84 (1992): 438–42.

Press, R. J., et al. "The Effect of Chromium Piccolinate on Serum Cholesterol and Apolipoprotein Fractions on Human Subjects." *The Western Journal of Medicine* 152, no. 1 (January 1990).

Prior, J. C. "Progesterone as a Bone-Tropic Hormone." *Endocrine Reviews* 11 (1990): 386–98.

Rall, L., et al. "Vitamin B-6 and Immune Competence." *Nutrition Reviews* 51, no. 8 (1993): 217–25.

Regelson, W., and Colman, C. *The Superhormone Promise.* New York: Simon & Schuster, 1996.

Salmi, H. A., et al. "Effect of Silymarin on Chemical, Functional and Morphological Alterations of the Liver." *Scandinavian Journal of Gastroenterology* 17 (1982): 517–21.

Sand, M., et al. "A Controlled Trial of Selegiline, Alpha Tocopherol, or Both as a Treatment for Alzheimer's Disease." *The New England Journal of Medicine* 336, no. 17 (April 24, 1997): 1216–22.

Satyavata, G. V. "Guggulipid: A Promising Hypolipidemic Agent from Gum Guggul (Commiphora Wightii.)" *Economic and Medicinal Plant Research* 5 (1991): 48–81.

Schenker, S., et al. "Polyunsaturated Lecithin and Alcoholic Liver Disease: A Magic Bullet?" *Alcoholism: Clin. Exp. Res.* 18 (1994): 1286–88.

Seddon, J., et al. "Dietary Carotenoids, Vitamins A, C, and E, and Advanced Age Related Macular Degeneration." *Journal* of the American Medical Association 272, no. 18 (1994): 1413–20.

Seddon, J. H., et al. "The Use of Vitamin Supplements and the Risk of Cataract Among U.S. Male Physicians." American Journal of Public Health 84, no. 5 (May 1994): 788–92.

Shansugasundaram, E. R. B., et al. "Use of Gymnema Sylvestre Leaf Extract in the Control of Blood Glucose in Insulin-Dependent Diabetes Mellitus." Journal of Ethnopharmacology 30 (1990): 281–94.

Sikora, R., et al. "Ginkgo Biloba Extract in the Therapy of Erectile Dysfunction." Journal of Urology 141 (1989): 141–88A.

Simopoulos, A. "Omega-3 Fatty Acids in Health and Disease and in Growth and Development." American Journal of Clinical Nutrition 54 (1991): 438–63.

Singh, Y. N. "Kava: An Overview." Journal of Ethnopharmacology 37, vol. 1 (1992): 13–45.

Sperduto, R. H., et al. "The Linxian Cataract Study: Two Nutrition Intervention Trials." Archives of Ophthalmology 111 (September 1993): 1246–53.

Stanko, R. T., et al. "Body Composition, Energy Utilization, and Nitrogen Metabolism with a 4.25 MJ/d Low-energy Diet Supplemented with Pyruvate." American Journal of Clinical Nutrition 56 (1992): 630–35.

Stephens, N. G., et al. "Randomized Controlled Trial of Vitamin E in Patients with Coronary Disease: Cambridge Heart Antioxidant Study (CHAOS)." The Lancet 347, no. 9004 (March 23, 1996): 781–86.

Teel, R. W., et al. "Antimutagenic Effects of Polyphenolic Compounds." Cancer Letter 66, no. 2 (September 30, 1992): 107–223.

Van Scott, E. J., et al. "Alpha Hydroxyacids: Therapeutic Potentials." The Canadian Journal of Dermatology 1 (November/ December 1989): 108–12.

Varma, S. "Scientific Basis for Medical Therapy of Cataracts by Antioxidants." American Journal of Clinical Nutrition 53 (1991): 335S–345S.

Yuji, M., et al. "Hypocholesterolemic Effect of Chitosan in Adult Males." *Bioscience Biotechnology Biochemistry* 5 (May 1995): 786–90.

Zhang, X., et al. "Protective Effects of Nicotinic Acid on Disturbance of Memory Retrial Induced by Cerebral Ischemia-Reperfusion in Rats." *Chin. J. Pharm. Tox.* 10 (1996): 178–80.

Zuchrua Zakay-Rones, Mumcuoglu M., et al. "Inhibition of Several Strains of Influenza Virus In Vitro and Reduction of Symptoms by an Elderberry Extract (Sambucus nigra) During an Outbreak of Influenza B Panama." *The Journal of Alternative and Complementary Medicine* 1 (1995): 361–69.

Index